CW00336305

MENIERE
IN THE KITCHEN

RECIPES
THAT
HELPED ME
GET OVER
MENIERE'S

PAGE ADDIE
UNITED KINGDOM AUSTRALIA

Copyright

Copyright©2013 by Meniere Man
All rights reserved. No reproduction, copy or transmission of this Publication may be made without written permission from the author. No paragraph of this publication may be reproduced, copied or transmitted. Save with written permission or in accordance with provisions of the Copyright, Designs and Patents Act 1988, or under the terms of any license permitting limited copying, issued by the Copyright Licensing Agency, The Author has asserted his right to be identified as the author of this work in accordance with the Copyright, Design and Patents Act 1988

Meniere Man In The Kitchen. Recipes that Helped Me Get Over Meniere's. ISBN 978-0-9928114-19 is published by Page Addie Press United Kingdom, BIC Subject category: VFJB A catalogue record for this book is available from Australian National Library. 1. meniere's disease. 2. meniere. 3. vertigo. 4. dizziness. 5. low sodium. 6. inner ear. 7. disease symptoms. 8 vestibular problems. 9. vertigo symptoms. 10 causes of vertigo. 11. imbalance in ear. 12. what is vertigo. 13 low salt diet. 14 coping with vertigo.

Disclaimer: Neither the Author of Publisher aim to give professional advice to the individual reader. The suggestions in this book are based on the experience of the Author only and are not intended to replace consultation with a doctor and/or dietician where health matters are concerned. Meniere's disease requires medical supervision as do all other health issues. Neither the Author or Publisher shall be responsible or liable for any injury, damage, loss arising from information or suggestions in this book as the opinions expressed are entirely derived from the Author's personal experience and the book expresses and represents the personal view of the Author. Every effort has been made to provide accurate website addresses and complete information at the date of publication, however exact measurements and cooking times are dependent on the quality of ingredients, the varying temperatures of kitchen equipment, therefore the readers commonsense is the best guide to compensate for such variables. The Author and the Publisher take no responsibility for individual health issues or specific allergies or allergy, known or otherwise, that needs specific medical supervision, or any adverse reaction to any ingredient specified, or adverse reactions to the recipes contained in this book. The recipes are chosen by the experience of the Author and are not advocated as a cure for Meniere's disease, but are based on the Author's personal experience and represents the Authors personal views on healthy eating as part of an overall plan to improve health, as experienced by the Author only. The recipes in this book and advice given are published for general interest for the reader only and are not intended to take the place of medical guidelines and recommendations by medical professionals.

MENIERE MAN
IN THE KITCHEN

RECIPES
THAT
HELPED ME
GET OVER
MENIERE'S

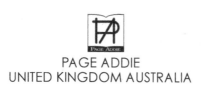

PAGE ADDIE
UNITED KINGDOM AUSTRALIA

DEDICATED TO SUE
*FOR YOUR CONSTANT LOVE AND SUPPORT THROUGH A
TIME OF MENIERE'S AND BEYOND.*

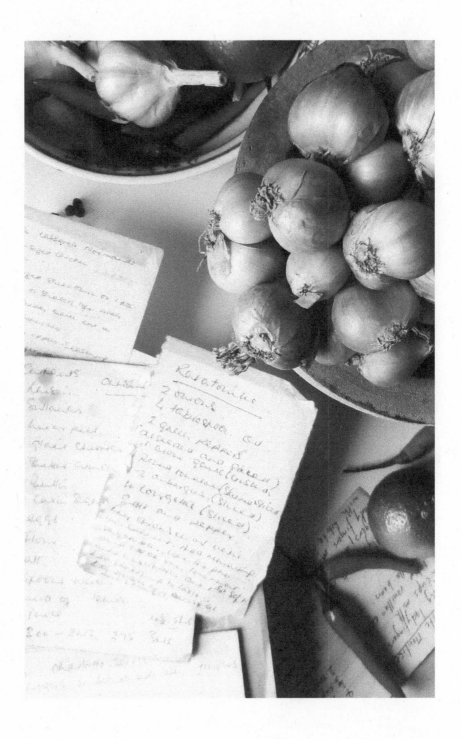

CONTENTS

ABOUT
MENIERE MAN'S
KITCHEN

YOU ARE WHAT YOU EAT

I believe diet played a key factor in helping me get over Meniere's. It wasn't until my diagnosis of Meniere's disease that I made significant changes to my diet.

I loved all the bad foods, the salted and the caffeinated; salami, dill pickles, ham, bacon, a double shot of espresso. In fact, the whole check list, of what not to eat, when you have Meniere's, were my favorites.

As a Meniere sufferer, making the right food choices is an important decision. It can make the difference between you having a vertigo attack or not. But there's more. I believe you need to do more than just leave salt out of your meals. Just reducing your salt intake is not enough to get you over Meniere's. Everyone agrees that reducing daily sodium intake should be part of your Meniere management plan. But you can do so much more than just throwing away the salt shaker.

To help yourself get over Meniere's, eating nutritional healing foods is a must. The healthier you eat, the better you become. This is what *Meniere Man In The Kitchen* is all about. Looking back, low salt plus eating healthily, were both major factors in my full recovery from Meniere's. So when people ask me for one of my low salt recipes, I always give it to them. Like all the best things in life, a good recipe gets better, the more it is shared.

Meniere Man In The Kitchen, is a collection of our family's favorite low salt recipes. In our recipes we don't count salt grams, but we don't add salt and we eliminate hidden salts. This book is about the love of food and not about counting salt grams. I initially tried counting grams but it become such a stressful, tedious exercise, that it took the romance and joy out of eating. Our recipes are so delicious you won't even miss the salt.

As you cook, you'll get to know some of the basic nutritional values of the ingredients. If you are not already eating a low salt diet for Meniere's, your taste buds will need to adapt a little to the taste of less salt. You may see recipes listed with spices and herbs you haven't tried. So this will be a new culinary adventure in taste. Just as turmeric and saffron were for me. Salt is just one kind of seasoning. Nature has a store cupboard of herbs and spices.

If you are already eating a low salt diet, then these recipes will make a welcome addition to your recipe books. I've found that you can never have enough recipe books in your kitchen.

Along with this book, and any other cookbook for that matter, you should have a pencil. It's a key ingredient.

With a pencil, you make notes and add your own thoughts and ideas. In this way all the recipes evolve and when people ask you, as they will, to share your low salt recipe, you can give them your culinary creation.

My recipes remind me of people and places; they are also a part of my healing journey. We now cook as a family, buying fresh produce in season, tasting everything, adjusting flavors and marrying ingredients without salt. It's my great pleasure to invite you to join us at our family table. Enjoy!

WHY SALT IS THE BAD BOY OF FOOD

Before I was diagnosed with Meniere's, my weekend was not complete without tucking into a big breakfast. Let's say you start the day with a full English or American breakfast. The 100gms of crispy bacon, more if you sneaked a few rashers while you were grilling it - contains 1021mg/ sodium. The two fried or scrambled farm eggs 148mg/ sodium, butter 826mg/sodium, two slices of toast 500mg/ sodium, two small grilled tomatoes 130 mg/sodium and a serving of baked beans 436 mg/sodium. The grand total for Sunday breakfast is 3061 mg/sodium.

Maintaining a sodium intake below 2000mg is a matter of making the right food choices. That's not to say you won't ever be able to eat a hearty cooked breakfast again with all your favorites, but if you are suffering with acute Meniere's symptoms, then salt is something you need to pay attention to. A heavily salted meal is something that puts you at risk of a vertigo attack. It's a recognized trigger.

The inner ear, when healthy, has its own independent regulatory fluid system, separate from the rest of the body. Consequently it is not affected by any chemical or blood fluid dynamics of the body's fluid system. When you have Meniere's, the vertigo attacks degenerate and destroy the healthy function of the inner ear which results in the loss of the inner ear's independent fluid function. This results in the inner ear's fluid volume and chemical concentration being subject to the rest of the body's fluid/blood system. Any fluctuation of the body's blood/fluid volume and chemical make-up can cause symptoms in the ear, such as the sensation of fullness, tinnitus, dizziness, imbalance and vertigo.

The inner ear is bathed in a very specific concentration of sodium and potassium. Now that the inner ear is no longer independent, if you change this delicate balance, by eating food high in salt (sodium) you will have a delivery of concentrated sodium solution into the inner ear. This results in an imbalance of sodium and potassium concentration. Then the inner ear desperately tries to balance the concentration levels by diluting the sodium with water. This, in turn, expands one of the compartments, so the separating membrane becomes extended. It ruptures and you have a Meniere vertigo attack.

So how much salt can you have? The body needs some salt, you can't live without some salt and that is a scientific fact. A low salt diet is 400-1000mg of salt a day. A normal salt diet is 1100-3300mg a day. A high salt diet is 4000-6000mg a day.

Maintaining a sodium intake below 1000mg a day takes effort. There is no need to be afraid of salt, you just need to control your intake. So the aim of a low sodium diet is to move the regulation system towards the lowest point of its range without pushing it to its limit and causing the actual sodium levels in the body to fail. If the low salt diet is taken to extremes, it can have an adverse reaction. Extremely low levels would need to be monitored by a doctor.

It's not just about salt you can see. There is hidden salt in many products, even the daily loaf of bread and tomato sauce. Read the food labels on cans and packets. The amount of salt is listed as sodium. Read the labels and compare sodium content. The difference can be huge. Buy the lowest sodium content on every item. Avoid salty foods such as processed meats and fish, pickles, relish, sauces especially soy sauce, salted nuts, chips and processed snack foods. Pretzels 1680mg/sodium per 100grams, potato chips up to 1000mg /sodium a portion. Foods that come in a tin or packet or ready cooked, like spaghetti sauce in a jar or dried soup in a packet, are usually high in salt. Beef and chicken stock cubes have 24,000mg of sodium per 100 grams. Dried beef 4,300 mg/sodium. Look for products that have the lowest sodium content, based on the amount you eat. You will see the nutritional box on the packet or tin. Many high sodium products such as tomato sauce show low sodium values because the sodium is based on small sodium portions. Many food manufacturers are already producing low salt products such as salt reduced baked beans, sodium reduced tuna fish and low salt feta cheese. Read the labels carefully before you buy. Avoid cooking with salt or adding salt to the cooking pot.

Talk to family about a low salt nutritious diet because it is not just about you; a low salt nutritious diet is healthier for everyone, because it reduces the risk of heart disease, strokes, high blood pressure and many other medical conditions.

REGENERATIVE FOODS

Adrenal Support

Your adrenals are two small glands that lie just above each kidney. When you have been overworking, under physical and physiological stress, your adrenals get exhausted and you feel run down. Having frequent vertigo attacks and generally coping with Meniere's disease symptoms puts you mentally and physically under stress. So it is important to give your adrenal glands support by eating foods that support and replenish adrenals. Vitamin C, Vitamin A and CoQ10 help reduce stress on the adrenals. Red meat, fats, sugar and white flour stress the adrenals. Foods that support adrenals are asparagus, leafy green vegetables, almonds, flax-seed, molasses, pumpkin seeds, whole grains, wheatgerm, blueberries, coconut, grapefruit, figs, prunes, lemons, oranges, strawberries, tuna and salmon.

Nerve Support.

Essential Oils: EFA's or Essential Fatty Acids are important in reducing inflammation and assisting nerve transmission. The body cannot make EFA's so they need to be obtained through diet. Good sources of EFA are borage oil, oil of primrose, nuts, seeds, fish, walnut and olive oil. Another good oil is Omega-3, found in fish, especially cold water oily fish like mackerel, herring, tuna, salmon and sardines. If you don't like fish, you can supplement your diet with cold pressed flax seed oil. The LSA recipe (further in this book) is a good one, linseed is another name for flax-seeds. Omega-9 fatty acid is found in avocado, almonds and olive oil, raw unprocessed oils, cold pressed oils such as cold pressed extra virgin oil.

Immune Boosters

Antioxidant foods help support the immune system because they help to stop free radicals from rampaging and damaging your system. Foods containing antioxidants are fresh fruits, berries, vegetables, barley, yogurt and garlic. You will find recipes with those ingredients in this book for that reason.

Plant Sterols

Eating well to get well involves using anti-inflammatory foods in your diet. Plant sterols are anti-inflammatory vegetable fats that improve circulation to the head and inner ear. Plant sterols are known to alleviate some symptoms of Meniere's disease. Young green shoots of alfalfa, mung beans and cress are rich in plant sterols

VITAMIN RICH FOODS

A low salt diet rich in vitamins and minerals will make a significant difference to your health. The more you understand the importance of minerals and vitamins for your general well-being, the more you'll be able to help yourself to obtain optimum health. You can take additional vitamin supplements in a daily and three monthly vitamin regime as outlined in *Meniere Man Let's Get Better*.

Vitamin A

Boosts the immune system. Found in dark green leafy, broccoli, vegetables, orange and yellow vegetables such as pumpkin and carrots, fish, eggs and milk.

Vitamin C

Vitamin C supports the kidneys, liver and immune system. Vitamin C is found in strawberries, blackberries, oranges, lemons, salad greens, avocado and grapefruit.

Vitamin E

Promotes healing and is a powerful antioxidant. Good sources are almonds, nuts, eggs, cold-pressed vegetable oils, grains.

Vitamin B2, B5, B12

B vitamins B6, B2, B5, and B12 are proven to assist the nervous system helping reduce stress, depression, relieve tension, pick up energy and assist nerve regeneration. Good sources are eggs, nuts, legumes, whole grains, spinach, fish, wheatgerm, peas, beans, seafood, and grains.

Calcium

May support the cochlear bone by preventing bone depletion. Good sources are broccoli, kelp, yogurt, almonds and green vegetables.

Magnesium

Helps with fatigue, depression and insomnia. Found in figs, whole grains, dried apricots, nuts, seeds and fish.

Manganese

Helps the nervous system. Good sources are egg yolks, nuts seeds, blueberries and avocado.

Zinc

Strengthens the immune system and improves cognitive function. Good sources of zinc are fish, eggs, legumes, pumpkin seeds, whole grain, wheat germ and bran.

Selenium

Keeps blood vessels healthy and improves the immune system. Good sources are seafood, salmon, tuna, garlic and Brazil nuts.

Chromium

Helps control cholesterol levels in the blood. Good sources are potatoes, grains, wheat germ.

Potassium

Helps maintain the fluid balance in the body. Good sources are potatoes, avocados, raisins, nuts, legumes, dairy products and fish.

Iron

Supports the nervous system. Good sources are beets, asparagus, figs, raisins and molasses.

THE HEALTHY KITCHEN STORE CUPBOARD

Substitute foods which are not so healthy for you and replace for foods which are naturally good for you and low in salt.

Salt

Replace with: kelp has natural iodine which gives a natural saltiness to food without the high sodium of table salt so it makes a good substitute in a low salt diet. Available in flakes, granules, dried and powder.

Cornstarch

Replace with arrowroot from the arrowroot plant.

Phosphate baking powder

Phosphate baking powder has a high sodium content Replace with low salt tartrate baking powder or low-sodium baking powder.

Double acting baking powder

Replace with low salt aluminum-free baking powder.

Baking soda

Replace with low-sodium aluminum-free baking powder (use two parts baking powder in place of one part soda for baking muffins, cookies, cakes and breads).

White sugar

Replace with raw sugar or a dark sugar; or raw honey, 1/2 cup of honey = 1 cup of white sugar (reduce the amount of liquid in the recipe by 1/4 of a cup and add an extra 3 tbsp of flour). Use pure maple syrup, fruit juices, purees, applesauce, mashed bananas, apple juice concentrate in recipes.

1 cup of white sugar = 1/2 cup apple juice concentrate.
1 cup of raw sugar = 1 cup of palm sugar.

Soft drinks

Replace with hot iced fruit teas, herbal teas, fruit juice, vegetable juice, mineral water (non-carbonated, low/sodium).

Chicken stock cubes

Replace with one cup of no-salt chicken broth made from chicken bones simmered one hour in water with vegetables and strained. You can freeze this in small, usable portions. Or use commercially prepared no-salt stock.

Beef bouillon cubes

Replace with home-made beef stock. Take beef marrow bones and roast them in the oven 200 degrees C for 30 minutes. Add water to the pan to take up the released juices. Place juice from pan and bones into a soup pot. Add vegetables such as carrots and onions to flavor the stock. Cover bones with 1 liter of water and simmer bones and vegetables, lid off, for one hour on low heat. Cool and strain.

Garlic powder

Replace with 1 clove of garlic crushed. Make a garlic paste. Roast the whole head of garlic in the oven until it softens to a paste. Use the paste in soups, vegetables, sandwiches and soups instead of garlic powder. Keep in the fridge.

Steak seasonings, barbecue seasonings

Replace with home made seasonings.

Italian seasoning - marjoram, basil, oregano, thyme, rosemary. Make an Italian spice mixture to add to marinades. Place 2 tbsp of black or white pepper in a grinder. Add 2 tsp dried marjoram, and 2 tsp of dried basil and 2 tsp dried oregano, 1 tsp thyme, 1 tsp rosemary. Grind all together and keep in an airtight jar in the fridge.

French seasoning - marjoram, rosemary, thyme, bay-leaf. Place 2 tbsp of black or white pepper in a grinder. Add 2 tsp cloves and 2 tsp of nutmeg and 1 tsp of powdered ginger. Grind all together and keep in an airtight jar.

English seasoning - rosemary, parsley, thyme and

sage. Place 2 tbsp of black or white pepper in a grinder. Add 2 tsp dried rosemary leaves and 2 tsp of dried thyme and 1 tsp of sage leaves and 2 tsp parsley flakes. Grind all together and keep in an airtight jar in the fridge.

Asian seasoning - ginger, fennel, star anise, pepper. Place 2 tbsp of black or white pepper in a grinder. Add 2 tsp ginger and 2 tsp of dried fennel and 1 tsp of star anise. Grind all together and keep in an airtight jar in the fridge.

For all-purpose seasoning - Replace salt with dried vegetables such as sun-dried tomatoes, garlic, onions, herbs, vinegars and kelp for seasoning.

Peanut butter

Replace with a no-salt brand.

Canned and packet soups

Replace with salt-free home-made meat, chicken, vegetable, fish broths and soups made from bones, herbs and vegetables.

Canned vegetables

Replace with raw, fresh or no-salt frozen/canned vegetables.

Dried fruits

Commercial dried fruits, apples, prunes, raisins, apricots and cranberries contain preservative. Replace with fruits which are organically grown and dried without preservative.

White flour

Replace with organic unbleached white flour, whole-meal, corn, rye, oat flour, buckwheat, rice flour. Avoid all white processed food products such as commercial cakes and biscuits.

Black tea and iced tea

Replace with green tea such as jasmine tea, fruit tea, spice and herb teas sweetened with a little honey.

Caffeinated coffee

Replace with quality brand of water processed decaffeinated coffee. If you have been drinking a lot of tea and coffee, substitute other beverages slowly to avoid a caffeine headache! Start with lemon juice in water each morning and then replace one cup of coffee or tea for a herbal tea.

Cereal

Most commercial cereals have excessive amounts of salt and sugar. Replace with oats and home-made granola and muesli.

Jam and jellies

Commercial jams are loaded with sugar. Replace with home-made fruit spread. Cut up the fruit of your choice, apples, peaches, nectarines, mangoes or berries. Puree them in a food processor, adding a little honey if they are tart. You can add lemon or lime juice and spices such as cardamom or cinnamon. Place the pureed fruit in a greased, flat baking dish and bake in a very low oven 150 degree C until thick, for 2-4 hours. Keep in a jar in the fridge.

Quick fruit puree - follow the recipe above but cook over low heat in a saucepan with a little honey or maple syrup to make a honey fruit or maple fruit jam. Prune jam - cook dried prunes in a little water and orange juice and a cinnamon stick. Remove cinnamon stick. Cool and puree to make prune jam.

Sweetened yogurt

Replace with plain yogurt (preferably organic or home-made) sweeten with honey and a teaspoon of vanilla, apple sauce with cinnamon, maple syrup, apricot nectar, peach nectar, stewed dried apricots, prunes, peaches, pineapple, apple fruit concentrate, muesli and granola, almonds and honey.

Canned beans and spaghetti

Replace with cooked beans without salt.

Cheeses, hard cheeses, parmesan and cheese spreads

Replace with no-salt cottage cheese, no-salt ricotta or soft tofu. Make your own no-salt cheese. Take 2 cups of fresh plain unsweetened acidophilus yogurt and chop your favorite herbs, chives, parsley, basil and mix until smooth then wrap the yogurt in a clean damp cotton muslin cloth. Suspend the "yogurt" above a bowl overnight and the juices will drain from the yogurt leaving a soft cheese in the morning. Chill and serve with crackers or bread, pita wraps or salads.

Anchovies, salted herrings

Replace with fresh white fish, tinned low salt tuna, fresh salmon.

Meats, smoked, pickled

Replace corned beef, gravy, ham, salami, bologna, meat pastes and pate with fresh turkey, chicken, lamb, beef, pork.

Nuts, salted, roasted

Replace with unsalted popcorn, fresh raw nuts, pine nuts, pumpkin seeds, sunflower seeds.

Salted potato crisps, pretzels

Replace with home-made crisps using very thinly sliced potatoes or sweet potato. Place on an oven tray and drizzle with olive oil. Sprinkle with black pepper. Bake in a 200 degree C oven until golden brown and crisp.

MEASUREMENTS

OVEN TEMPERATURE CONVERSION CHART

(DEGREE) F	(DEGREE) C
200	100
225	110
250	120
275	140
300	150
325	160
350	180
375	190
400	200
425	220
450	230
475	240

COOKING MEASUREMENTS

Liquids

1 tsp equals 5mls
1 tbsp equals 20mls
4 cups equals 1 liter
1/2 cup equals 125mls

Weights

32oz equals 1 kilogram
16oz equals 500grams
8 oz equals 250grams
7 oz equals 220 grams
6oz equals 185 grams
5 oz equals 155 grams
4 oz equals 125 grams
3 oz equals 90 grams
2 oz equals 60 grams
1 oz equals 30 grams

I cup = Equivalent

1 cup oats = 100 g
1 cup corn flour = 190 g
1 cup whole nuts = 150g
1 cup chopped nuts = 125 g
1 cup unbleached plain flour = 155g
1 cup wholemeal flour = 155g
1 cup shredded coconut = 90 g
1 cup raw sugar = 250 g

20 NUTRIENT RICH SNACK IDEAS

1 Celery sticks filled with unsalted peanut butter.
2 Celery sticks filled with unsalted cottage cheese.
3 Cottage cheese with unsweetened pineapple.
4 Plain yogurt. Add passion fruit and honey. Or any fresh fruit, stewed dried prunes, stewed dried apricots. Sprinkle with LSA.
5 Plain yogurt with LSA and honey.
6 Half a pita bread filled with all or some of the following: sprouts, salad greens, sliced tomato, shredded carrots, grated beetroot, and slices of avocado.
Add a small tin of no-salt tuna or salmon.
Add a hardboiled egg. Add no-salt cottage cheese. Dress with your choice of no-salt salad dressing.
7 Six almonds and half an apple.
8 Pita bread with leftover meatloaf or burgers, tomato salsa with salad green.

9 Rye bread with avocado, salad greens and homemade mango chutney.

10 Soup of the day or broth.

11 Fruit smoothie made with blended fruits and ice; fruit and yogurt with ice.

12 Vegetable juices or fruit and vegetable combined juice such as carrot and apple.

13 Coconut water. Add to fruit to make a smoothie. Drink a coconut a day during times of acute vertigo attacks. Coconut water and flesh have powerful healing enzymes.

14 Essene bread and mashed banana.

15 A handful of pumpkin or sunflower seeds.

16 Seed and grain crackers (see recipe) topped with salsa, humus or chutney.

17 Fruit muffins.

18 Nut muffins.

19 Carrot cake.

20 Soup, broth and healthy cracker.

REGENERATIVE RECIPES

BREAKFAST

Bircher Muesli

Ingredients

1 cup apple juice

1 cup fat reduced thick yogurt

1/2 cup blanched almonds, chopped

1/4 cup sesame seeds

1/2 cup hazelnuts, chopped

3 cups rolled oats

1 1/2 cups dried apple or freshly grated apple

2/3 cup sultanas or raisins (organic)

2 tsp cinnamon

Method

Heat the oven to 180 degrees C.
Toast the seeds and nuts for 5-8 minutes. Take
care not to burn. Toss with the oats, sultanas

and cinnamon.
Place 2 cups in a bowl and add one cup of
apple juice. Mix together and add the yogurt.
Cover and refrigerate overnight and serve with
grated apple or dried apple.

Variations

Substitute raisins or sultanas for dried
blueberries, cherries or blueberries.
Substitute the apples for fresh stone fruit such
as peaches, apricots, pears or stewed fruits
such as plums. Or fresh berries in season.

Health benefits of this recipe.
*Fresh berries are one of nature's super foods having
potent immune power. High in antioxidants are apricots,
apples, kiwi fruit, all types of seeds and nuts.*

French Crepes

Ingredients

1 cup plain flour

1 tbsp unsalted butter, melted

1 whole egg

1 egg yolk

1 cup of milk

Method

Beat all ingredients together until smooth.
Leave batter to rest for 30 minutes.
Melt a little butter in a crepe or frying pan.
Pour batter in a thin stream. Keep the crepes
thin. Serve with maple syrup, berries, lemon or
orange juice and raw sugar.

Variation.

Slice fresh mango or banana or thinly sliced
pineapple onto the batter for tropical pancakes.
Fill the pancakes with mushrooms and chicken
in a white sauce and bake in a 190 degrees C
oven for savory pancakes.

Health benefits of this recipe
*Eggs and milk are high in protein, zinc, B and E
vitamins.*

Maple and Hazelnut Granola

Ingredients

3 cups rolled oats

1/2 cups chopped hazelnuts

1/4 cup wheat germ

1/2 cup maple syrup

2/3 cup dried peaches, chopped

Method

Heat oven to 160 degrees C.

Place grains in baking tray on non-stick paper.

Drizzle over maple syrup and bake 20 minutes.

Stir once. Cook until toasted and golden.

Toss with peaches and allow to cool.

Store in an airtight container in the fridge or freezer.

Serves 4-6 people. Keeps for a month

Variation

Use dried apricots, dried apples, and dried pears instead of peaches.

Substitute hazelnuts for almond, walnuts, pecans etc.

Add cinnamon and spices.

Use oats with other grains and seeds added.

Substitute honey for maple syrup.

Oats can be served hot or cold in granola and muesli. They add a nutty flavor when added to baking.

Health benefits of this recipe.
Oats are high in protein, and fiber and particularly high in vitamin E and vitamin B and calcium. Oats are known to lower cholesterol.

Very Berry Muesli

Ingredients

1/2 cup slivered almonds

2 tbsp sesame seeds

3 cups rolled oats

2 cups fresh squeezed orange juice or apple juice

1 1/2 cups plain low fat yogurt

1 red apple, grated

1 tsp cinnamon

fresh or frozen berries

Method

Toast almonds and sesame seeds in an 180 degrees C oven for 4 minutes. Cool.
Combine oats, red apple and cinnamon with orange or apple juice. Add yogurt and mix together. Leave overnight in a bowl in the fridge.
Serve topped with your choice of fresh seasonal berries: strawberries, blueberries, raspberries. Or use thawed frozen berries lightly warmed with a little honey to make a berry compote.
Serves 6.

Health benefits of this recipe.

Apple juice is high in minerals. It has cleansing properties and helps reduce internal inflammation. Apple juice is good for helping liver function. Orange juice is high in vitamin C.

Steve's Pancakes

Ingredients

4 cups unbleached flour

4 cups warm milk (lukewarm)

1 tbsp sugar

1 tbsp dried baker's yeast

1 tsp low-sodium baking powder

4 eggs

olive oil - light

maple syrup

lemon

caster sugar

Method

Add sugar to 1/4 cup of the lukewarm milk. Add yeast to this. Mix and leave in a warm place until it bubbles.

Add the rest of the warm milk and flour. Stir and cover with a towel for an hour. Add 4 eggs and baking powder. Mix well.

Cook in a hot fry pan using a small amount of olive oil to stop the pancakes sticking. Serve with maple syrup and berries or lemon and caster sugar.

Serves 6-8

Variation

These are American style pancakes and this recipe makes a good sized batch ideal for a family breakfast. Milk and eggs make this a high protein breakfast.

Drizzle maple syrup or honey, or a little raw sugar and lemon juice over the cooked pancakes. Berries lightly cooked with a little honey or raw sugar make a great warm syrupy topping.

Sophie's French Toast

Ingredients

1 loaf of brioche bread or a any slightly sweet
bread or plain 9 inch loaf

1/2 cup unsalted butter

5 eggs, large

1 1/2 cups light cream

1 tsp vanilla essence

1 tsp Grand Marnier (optional)

Method

Melt butter in a small saucepan with sugar. Stir
over moderate heat until smooth and pour this
into a 13 x 9 x 2 inch baking dish. Cut crusts off
the loaf of bread and make six one inch cubes
of bread. Arrange bread in one layer.
Whisk eggs, vanilla, Grand Marnier and light
cream, until combined. Pour over the bread in
the dish. Chill all in the fridge for 8 hours and
up to one day before baking.
Bake in a 180 degrees C oven uncovered for
35 minutes - or until puffed up and golden.
Serve immediately. Serves 4-6.

Variation

Substitute fruit bread for the brioche.
This recipe is from our friend Sophie who
lives in South West France. It's a deliciously
decadent version of French toast.

Yogurt with Watermelon

Ingredients

3 cups of thick fat-reduced yogurt

1/4 cup of liquid honey

1 tsp of rosewater

pistachio nuts, unsalted, shelled and chopped

watermelon deseeded and roughly chopped

red or pink rose petals, washed and dried

Method

Mix yogurt and honey together and add rosewater. Place watermelon in a bowl. Pour over yogurt and decorate with pistachio nuts and rose petals. Serves 4-6

Health benefits of this recipe.
High in iron, magnesium, potassium, zinc and C and E.

Linseed, Sunflower, Almond Mix

Ingredients

Equal quantities of the following:
linseed
whole almonds with skins
sunflower kernels

Method

Grind up in a clean coffee grinder or food processor. Mix together and store in the fridge or freezer. Use to sprinkle on yogurt, cereals and salads or eat a dessert spoon as a nutritious snack rich in essential oils. Add to muffins, breads and cookies.

Health benefits of this recipe.
Almonds are called the king of nuts because they are higher in calcium and fiber than any other nut. High in potassium, magnesium and zinc. Sunflower seeds have a nutty flavor and contain vitamins, especially vitamin E, C and B's, plus calcium, potassium and zinc. Linseeds are rich in Omega-3's. This combination of nuts and seeds makes a great source of essential fatty acids.

ENTREES

Bruchetta

Ingredients

1 French loaf
4 vine ripe tomatoes
extra virgin olive oil
black pepper, freshly ground
2 cloves of garlic
basil leaves, finely shredded

Method

Finely chop the tomatoes. Place in a small bowl and add a drizzle of olive oil and a grind of pepper. Leave to stand 30 minutes at room temperature.
Slice bread thinly on an angle. Places slices on a baking sheet and carefully toast both sides.

As soon as the bread comes out of the oven, cut the clove of garlic and rub over the surface. Pour a little olive oil over each toast. Top with a tsp of tomato mixture on each of the toasts and add a few shreds of basil to garnish. Place on a serving platter.

Serves 6

Health benefits of this recipe.

Basil acts as an immune stimulant and is high in vitamin A, vitamin C, calcium and iron, potassium, manganese, magnesium and B vitamins.

Steamed Pork Dumplings

Ingredients

3 dozen wonton wrappers (fresh or frozen)

Filling

200g lean pork chopped

100g prawns, peeled

1/3 cup water chestnuts, chopped

4 Chinese dried mushrooms, soaked 30 minutes in hot water, drained, stalks discarded

1 spring onion, chopped

1 tbsp fresh ginger, chopped

Method

Put filling ingredients into food processor and process to a course paste. Fill each wonton wrapper with 2 tbsp of filling. Place in middle of wrapper, wet on edge with water, fold over, crimp edges to seal filling inside. Steam in lightly oiled bamboo or metal steamer 10 - 15 minutes. Serve hot with dipping sauce of 2 tsp low salt light soy diluted with 1/2 teaspoon of warm water.

Serves 4-6

Health benefits of this recipe.
Water chestnuts are a good source of minerals such as zinc, iron, magnesium and potassium.

Rocky's Oysters

Ingredients

1 dozen large rock oysters, in shell - detach the
oysters and put back in shell
2 cloves of garlic, finely chopped
1 small fresh chili (optional)
1 tbsp fresh ginger, finely chopped
1 tbsp lemon grass, finely chopped
1 tbsp mint, finely chopped
vegetable oil
1/2 cup lime juice
3 tbsp sugar
freshly ground pepper
roast blanched peanuts, finely chopped

Method

Bring lime juice and sugar to the boil. Season
with pepper. Gently fry the garlic, chili, ginger
and lemon grass until aromatic. Stir in the
mint and add the oysters. Gently stir fry until
the oysters color. Put an oyster back in each
shell with some of the herbs. Spoon over the
hot lime sauce - sprinkle with peanuts. Serve
garnished with mint and lime halves.

Health benefits of this recipe.

Oysters are high in zinc and calcium. Mint helps relieve insomnia and nervous tension and is high in Vitamin A and Vitamin C. Chili stimulates the endorphins (the body's natural painkiller) and is a powerful antioxidant. Peanuts have calcium, iron, magnesium, potassium and zinc. Avoid completely if allergic to peanuts.

Delicious Mauritius Prawn Chutney

Ingredients

6 large fresh prawns

1 green chili (optional)

1 tbsp fresh ginger

4 spring onions

juice of 1 lemon

soy bean oil

unsalted butter

Method

Cook shelled prawns in a little butter. Take care not to overcook. Add with other ingredients into food processor. Add soy bean oil as you blend, just enough to make a chunky paste. It has a wonderful color. Serve in a bowl surrounded by your favorite low salt or no-salt crackers.

Health benefits of this recipe.

Onions have anti-inflammatory properties and act as a blood tonic. They contain magnesium, calcium, potassium, zinc, manganese, vitamin C, vitamin E and B vitamins. Soy oil is a good source of omega-3 essential fatty acids.

SOUPS

The Chilean Visitor's Gazpacho

Ingredients

1 kg acid-free tomatoes, chopped

1 cucumber, peeled, chopped

1 brown or red onion, peeled, chopped

1 red sweet pepper, seeded, chopped

6 cloves of garlic, peeled

3 tbsp red wine vinegar

2/3 cup extra virgin olive oil

croutons, chopped hardboiled egg, chopped chives

Method

Puree vegetables in a food processor or blender in small batches until smooth. Add some water if too thick. Strain through a medium mesh sieve. Discard seeds and skins. Pour half back into the food processor. Add vinegar and puree until smooth, slowly adding olive oil. Add the puree and vegetable mixture together. Chill overnight. Serve cold garnishes on top of each bowl: croutons, chopped hardboiled egg, chopped chives.

Vegetable Potassium Broth

Ingredients

4 cups water

1 medium potato, chopped including skin

1 cup carrots, sliced, unpeeled

1 cup celery, washed and chopped

1 cup of brown onions, washed, cut into
quarters, including skin

2 cloves of garlic, crushed including skin

white pepper, freshly ground, to taste

Method

Place vegetables in a saucepan, add water and
bring to boil. Lower heat, cover and simmer
for one hour. Remove from heat and strain the
vegetables from the broth. Serve in cup with
unsalted crackers.

Variation

Add all or any of the following to vary the flavor
depending what is in season.
2 cups of chopped beetroot, 1/2 a medium
cabbage, chopped, 1/2 a bunch of parsley.

Health benefits of this recipe.
This soup is high in potassium rich vegetables.

Consuelo's Green Soup

Ingredients

1 large bunch of watercress. Leaves only

4 potatoes, peeled and chopped

1 medium onion, chopped

2 cloves garlic, crushed

5 small pearl onions, chopped

5 shallots, peeled and chopped (optional)

1 bunch of spring onions, use white part for soup

green tops of spring onions for garnish, chopped

2 cups non-fat milk

1 cup no-salt/low salt chicken stock (homemade preferably)

white or black pepper to taste

fresh coriander (cilantro) to garnish

Method

Place all onions, potatoes and garlic in a soup pot and cover with milk. Bring to the boil and reduce heat to a low simmer. Simmer until the potatoes are cooked. Add leaves of watercress and cook for another few minutes. When cool enough, blend together to make a green soup. Reheat but take care not to boil. Serve with croutons and black or white pepper. Garnish with coriander and/or watercress leaves.

Health benefits of this recipe.
Watercress is high in vitamin C and contains powerful antioxidants.

Summer Pea and Mint Soup

Ingredients

6 cloves of garlic

large bunch of mint, washed

50g unsalted butter

2 tbsp olive oil

1 kg peas

1 liter of low salt chicken stock

pepper

500ml Greek yogurt

Method

Finely chop the garlic and mint leaves. Melt the butter with olive oil in a large saucepan. Add the garlic and most of the mint and cook over a medium heat until golden brown. Add the peas and the chicken stock. Bring to boil. Liquidize using a hand blender until smooth. Season with pepper. When cool add 400 ml of yogurt and a few ice cubes to the soup. Serve out into 8 bowls. Top with yogurt and mint.

Health benefits of this recipe.
Peas are high in vitamin C so they help boost the immune system. Nutrient rich, green peas balance the fluid in the body and assist healthy cell function.

Spanish Lemon Soup

Ingredients

1 liter of home-made chicken stock
pepper
2 eggs
1 lemon, juiced
100g uncooked rice
garlic croutons made from French bread cut in
cubes and cooked in a little oil and garlic
1 bunch or Italian parsley, finely chopped

Method

Place stock in a soup pan. Bring the stock to
boil and add washed rice. Simmer over low
heat for 10 minutes until the rice is cooked.
Beat eggs with lemon juice and 1/4 of the
cooked stock and whisk. Add to the soup and
stir constantly until the soup thickens. Take
care not to boil. Take off the heat and serve
immediately with a bowl of chopped parsley
and garlic croutons.

Health benefits of this recipe.
*Lemons are high in vitamin C. They help to cleanse the
blood and liver and boost the immune system. Chicken
stock contains nutrients such as protein and calcium.*

Edgemoor Pumpkin Soup

Ingredients

1 kg pumpkin, cut into cubes

2 potatoes, peeled and chopped

1 onion, chopped

2 cloves of garlic, chopped

1 liter home-made chicken stock or (bought chicken broth - no-salt)

Method

Fry onion and garlic in 1 tbsp olive oil until transparent and soft. Add pumpkin and potato chunks and stir. Cover with chicken stock and simmer one hour on low heat. When cooked, cool. Blend until smooth and reheat. Add ground black pepper to taste.

Variation

Add juice of one orange. Add 1 tbsp grated fresh ginger. Substitute peeled and chopped carrots for the pumpkin.

Health benefits of this recipe.
Pumpkin helps fight infection and maintains fluid balance in the body.

Mum's Winter Vegetable Soup

Ingredients

2 onions, peeled and chopped

2 cloves garlic, crushed

5 celery stalks, washed and sliced

4 carrots, chopped

2 large potatoes, chopped

2 leeks, white part, sliced

1 cup pumpkin, chopped

pepper

olive oil

1 liter beef or chicken stock, no-salt - low salt,

parsley, chopped to garnish

Method

Fry onions and garlic in a little oil. Add the rest of the vegetables. Sauté until aromatic. Cover with stock. Simmer uncovered for one hour. Serve hot with bread, croutons and chopped parsley to garnish.

Variation

Vary the vegetables and add herbs of your choice. To make a hearty mid-winter soup, add meat or chicken, drained and rinsed white beans or brown lentils. To make a cream of vegetable soup, blend when cool and heat with a little milk. Do not boil.

Health benefits of this recipe.
Leeks are high in vitamin A, C and potassium.

Autumn Mushroom Soup

Ingredients

2-4 cups of assorted cultivated raw
mushrooms, washed and sliced
1 liter of low/salt no-salt chicken or vegetable
stock
5 brown shallots or 1/2 an onion, peeled and
chopped finely
1 potato, peeled and chopped
1 clove of garlic, crushed
olive oil
black pepper, ground
garlic bread croutons

Method

Sautee onions and garlic in a little oil on low
heat until transparent. Transfer to soup pot. Add
mushrooms, potato and stock. Bring to boil and
simmer on low heat for 30 minutes. When cool,
blend until smooth. Reheat gently and serve.
For garlic croutons, cut slices of day old French
bread into small cubes. Heat a little olive oil in a
pan. Add garlic and bread. Cook croutons until
crispy and brown. Serve on top of the soup.

Variation

Add 1/4 tsp of fresh or dried marjoram or 1/2 a bay leaf to the stock when cooking. Add a little milk when reheating to make a creamy soup. Add a tablespoon of yogurt and freshly chopped chives to serve.

Health benefits of this recipe.

Mushrooms stimulate the immune system, improve circulation, protect the liver and increase stamina.

Chicken and Sweet Pepper Soup

Ingredients

1 liter chicken stock

1 chicken breast

black or white pepper, freshly ground

2 red sweet peppers

2 yellow sweet peppers

Method

Place peppers on a tray in the oven and roast at 240 degrees C until brown, turning them until all the sides are brown. Place peppers in a food grade plastic bag and seal. Leave for 10 minutes, then place on a chopping board, saving the juice, peel the peppers and deseed them. Cut into long strips. Place the chicken breast in the stock and simmer 30 minutes or until the breast is cooked. Shred the chicken and add back to the pot. Heat the stock and add the peppers and their juice. Cook for five minutes on low heat and serve.

74

SALADS

Rusty's Market Mango Salad

Ingredients

4 ripe mangoes peeled and cut into thin strips.
2 carrots, peeled and cut into thin strips
1 tbsp extra virgin olive oil
1 lime, juiced
1 orange, juiced
coriander leaves, chopped
cracked black pepper

Method

Make a dressing with juice and oil. Add
coriander leaves and pepper.
Arrange mango and carrot strips on a serving
dish. Pour dressing over.

Health benefits of this recipe
Mangoes are very high in vitamin A, C and are high in fiber. The enzymes in mangoes help digestion. Mangoes help with circulation.

Potts Point Salad Nicoise

Ingredients

500g fresh green beans

1 red onion, cut into fine rings

1 cucumber, peeled and sliced thinly

5 fresh tomatoes, chopped

1 green bell pepper, sliced thinly

8 new potatoes, small

3 eggs

1 can low salt tuna fish in spring water, drained

cracked pepper

toasted garlic croutons

8 fresh basil leaves (optional)

extra virgin olive oil

Method

Cook green beans in boiling water and rinse under cold water. Drain. Boil potatoes and cut in half. Place vegetables on a serving dish. Top with fish. Cook eggs to soft boiled and spoon over the salad. Add a drizzle of olive oil, cracked pepper and garlic croutons and basil.

Variation

Use fresh fish such as grilled salmon or tinned

low salt salmon to make salmon Nicoise. Add drained artichokes, thinly sliced.

Health benefits of this recipe.

Green beans help with liver function and pancreas. Rich in fiber, iron, magnesium, potassium, zinc and vitamins C, E and B's. Potatoes are high in potassium.

Grilled Pepper Salad

Ingredients

4 red bell peppers

4 yellow bell peppers

olive oil

pepper

6 fresh basil leaves

Method

Heat oven to 200 degrees C. Place pepper on a baking tray and roast, turning twice until the skins turn brown. Take out of oven and seal in a food-safe plastic bag. Leave for 20 minutes. Then peel the skin and cut in half and remove the seeds. Save the juice. Add a little olive oil to the juice and freshly ground black pepper. Slice peppers into thin strips. Pour juices over as a dressing. Top with shredded fresh basil. Serve at room temperature.

Mushroom Salad

Ingredients

1 punnet of raw button mushrooms, washed
and sliced
1/2 tsp fresh marjoram or oregano, chopped
cracked pepper

Method

Place mushrooms in a bowl. Add cracked
pepper and chopped herbs. Add dressing, toss.
refrigerate 30 minutes before serving.

Dressing

6 tbsp safflower, extra virgin olive oil
3 tbsp wine or champagne vinegar
Place all ingredients in a screw top jar and
shake.

Health benefits of this recipe.
*Mushrooms are high in B vitamins, vitamin C and
potassium.*

Rocket and Orange Salad

Ingredients

2 oranges, peeled and sliced

2 tbsp orange juice

bag of rocket salad greens

2 tbsp pine nuts, toasted

2 tbsp walnut oil

mint leaves for garnish

Method

Toast pine nuts in a pan till golden. Mix orange juice with walnut oil. Place rocket and orange slices on a serving platter. Dress with orange and walnut dressing. Sprinkle with toasted pine nuts. Garnish with mint leaves.

Variations

Add 3 ripe avocado, sliced. Use lemon juice instead of orange juice. Use segments of grapefruit instead of oranges.

Health benefits of this recipe.
Pine nuts contain magnesium, potassium, zinc, iron and protein.

Warm Roasted Pear Salad

Ingredients

4 pears, sliced into wedges with skin on
bag of rocket salad greens
small bunch fresh rosemary leaves
2 tbsp olive oil
walnuts, toasted to garnish

Method

Heat oven to 180 degrees C. Place cut pears on a baking tray. Drizzle with olive oil and ground pepper and rosemary leaves (not stalks).
Roast in oven until crisp and brown but still firm. Place rocket on serving plate. Arrange warm pears. Sprinkle with toasted walnut halves.

Health benefits of this recipe.
Pears are rich in vitamin C, fiber and folate. Walnuts are high in potassium, magnesium and high in essential fatty acids. Rocket contains calcium, iron, fiber, potassium, zinc and magnesium as well as vitamin C, vitamin B's, folate, vitamin E and beta-carotene.

Easy Cabbage Pickle

Ingredients

1/2 red cabbage, finely shredded

1/2 green cabbage, finely shredded

1 tsp sea salt (to help extract the water from the cabbage)

1 tsp caraway seeds

1 tsp mustard seeds

Method

Place cabbages in a non reactive bowl. Add 1 tsp of salt. Mix for 2 minutes with your hands. Add the spices.

Place the cabbage into clean jars. Place a cabbage leaf on top of the mixture. Press down. Place a lid loosely on the jar. Leave at room temperature. Each day press down on the cabbage and replace the lid loosely. At the end of the third day, remove the cabbage leaf, tighten the lid and place in the fridge. Serve on crackers or with meats.

Health benefits of this recipe.
Cabbage helps the immune system and purifies the blood.

Green Mango Salad with Lime Prawns

Ingredients

1kg fresh prawns peeled and de-veined with tails

1 tbsp lime zest, shredded

2 tsp peanut oil

2 large green mangoes cut into thin strips

1/2 cup coriander leaves 1/2 cup mint leaves

1 cup bean sprouts

1/4 cup spring onions, thinly sliced

1 tbsp lime juice, fresh squeezed

3 tsp brown palm sugar, grated

Method

Mango salad: Combine mangoes, leaves, sprouts and spring onions. Dress with lime and sugar mixed together and a grind of black pepper. Lime prawns: cook prawns in peanut oil, and lime zest.

Place green mangoes salad on a plate and top with lime prawns.

Health benefits of this recipe.

Good source of protein, amino acids, potassium, magnesium, folate and vitamin C, and B's.

Summer Greek Salad

Ingredients

4 vine-ripened tomatoes, cut in chunks

1 green pepper, chopped

1 small cucumber, sliced thinly

1 red onion, sliced thinly into rings

1 bunch of parsley chopped

1 tsp fresh oregano, chopped

2 tbsp extra virgin olive oil

black pepper freshly ground

Method

Place all ingredients on a serving plate. Grind pepper over and drizzle with oil. Toss and serve.

Health benefits of this recipe.
Red onions, a blood tonic, anti-inflammatory properties.

Black Bean Salad with Limes

Ingredients

3 cans of black beans, rinsed and drained
1/2 cup of mild salsa
3 tbsp lime juice
1/2 purple onion, chopped
2 tbsp cilantro (coriander) chopped
1 red bell pepper, seeded and chopped
black pepper
1/4 cup extra virgin olive oil

Method

Combine all ingredients in a non-reactive container. Makes 8 cups. Store in the fridge.

Health benefits of this recipe.
Black beans are high in protein, fiber, iron, magnesium, potassium, zinc and B vitamins.

Easy Lettuce Salad

Ingredients

1 iceberg lettuce cut into six wedges

Dressing

1/3 cup olive oil

2 tbsp lemon juice

1/2 tsp caster (fine granulated sugar)

2 tsp fresh thyme, chopped

cracked black pepper

Method

Place all dressing ingredients in a small container. Shake dressing and pour over lettuce slices.

Variation

Use other fresh herbs such as oregano or basil. Substitute lime juice for lemon juice.

Health benefits of this recipe.

Iceberg lettuce is a good source of vitamin A, calcium, potassium, zinc, magnesium, vitamin C and vitamin B's as well as folate and amino acids.

Parsley and Mint Salad

Ingredients

120g bulgur wheat or cooked couscous

2 lemons, juiced and strained

4 tomatoes, diced

4 cloves of garlic, crushed and finely chopped

1 cup of fresh parsley, washed, leaves only

1 cup of fresh mint, washed, leaves only

2 tbsp extra virgin olive oil

Method

If using wheat, soak in cold water for ten minutes. Drain and squeeze water out.
Place in a bowl and add lemon juice and add extra virgin olive oil.
Add mint, parsley and garlic. Toss together.
Grind over black pepper.
Serve with wedges of lemon to garnish and tomatoes on the top.

Health benefits of this recipe.
Bulgur wheat contains fiber, choline, vitamin B's, vitamin E and iron. Parsley is high in vitamin C.

Avocado and Orange Salad

Ingredients

2 avocados, peeled and sliced

3 oranges, peeled and sliced into circles

cracked pepper

1 orange squeezed for dressing

1 tsp balsamic vinegar

2 tsp extra virgin olive oil

Method

Arrange oranges on a serving dish. Add avocado slices. Mix juice, balsamic and oil together. Add cracked black pepper. Pour over the oranges and avocado as a dressing and serve.

Avocado Dressing

Ingredients

2 avocados peeled

1 clove garlic

2 tsp lemon or lime juice

ground white pepper

1/2 cup plain unsweetened yogurt

Method

Mash avocados with garlic clove. Add lemon juice. Mix well. Add yogurt. Serves as a salad dressing, as a dressing for baked or boiled potatoes or as a dip.

Health benefits of this recipe.
Rich in vitamins B and D. Good for fatigue and nerves. Yogurt boosts the immune system and is high in protein, calcium, and potassium and B vitamins.

Diego's Avocado

Ingredients

3 avocados peeled

1-2 cloves garlic

2-3 tsp lemon or lime juice

4 tomatoes, chopped roughly

bunch of cilantro (fresh coriander)

chopped finely including roots

coriander leaves for garnish

tomato salsa

toasted cornbread broken into crisps

Method

Mash the avocados and add lemon or lime
juice. Add tomatoes and mix carefully through.
Add chopped cilantro and pepper. Pour into a
serving dish, top with tomato salsa. Surround
with corn chips for a dip, or serve on toasted
bread or in sandwiches with salad vegetables
and tuna.

Lime Mint Dressing

Ingredients

3/4 cup olive oil

1/4 cup fresh lime juice

1/4 tsp white pepper

1 tsp parsley, finely chopped

1 tsp mint, finely chopped

1 tsp chives, finely chopped

1 tsp French mustard

Method

Mix all ingredients together and beat with a cube of ice until it has the consistency of a medium cream sauce. Use for tossed salad.

Cucumber Salad with Yogurt Dressing

Ingredients

1 cucumber, chopped finely

1 small carton of reduced plain yogurt

white pepper, freshly ground

2 cloves of garlic, crushed

mint leaves, finely chopped, no stalk

extra virgin olive oil

toasted pita bread in wedges

Method

Make this salad just before serving.
Place yogurt into a bowl and add garlic, pepper.
Mix well. Add the cucumber pieces. Toss well.
Place in a serving dish and drizzle with a little
olive oil. Surround with toasted pita bread in
wedges.

Health benefits of this recipe.
Cucumbers are good for nerve function and are high in vitamin A.

Beetroot and Carrot salad

Ingredients

2 beetroots, washed, peeled and shredded

2 carrots, washed, peeled and shredded

2 stalks celery, chopped

1 apple, cut in small chunks

1 tbsp pinenuts, toasted

1 tbsp raisins

Method

Shred or grate the beetroot and carrot in a bowl together. Add apples and celery. Top with pinenuts and raisins. Serve with salad dressing.

Health benefits of this recipe.
Beetroot has a cleansing effect on the kidneys and liver. Beets are good for the blood.

Spinach and Egg Salad

Ingredients

Spinach, small leaf, washed and dried, stalks removed

2 eggs

olive oil

2 cloves garlic, crushed

French bread, 3 slices cut into cubes

black pepper, crushed

2 tbsp pinenuts, toasted

Dressing

3 tbsp balsamic vinegar,

6 tbsp extra virgin olive oil

Method

Place raw spinach in a serving bowl. Heat a little oil in a frying pan. Beat eggs and scramble in the pan. Remove and cool. Heat a little oil and fry garlic to flavor the oil. Add bread and cook until golden. Place eggs on spinach and top with bread croutons. Grind over black pepper. Dress with balsamic dressing.
Place oil and vinegar in a screw top container and shake.

Variations

Use toasted sunflower seeds instead of pine nuts.

Health benefits of this recipe.

Spinach is a powerful antioxidant that protects nerve cells. Spinach is rich in B vitamins and helps the body cope with stress. Pine nuts contain magnesium, zinc, potassium, protein and vitamins C, B's, A and essential fatty acids.

Asparagus and Parsley Salad

Ingredients

5 fresh asparagus spears, chop finely

1/4 cucumber, chopped finely

1/2 bunch parsley, chopped finely

2 stalks of celery, chopped finely

Method

Mix all ingredients in a bowl and top with dressing and serve.

Dressing

1/2 cup extra virgin olive oil

1/4 cup balsamic vinegar

1 tbsp liquid honey

1 tsp freshly chopped basil or parsley

black pepper, ground

Method

Place all dressing ingredients in a screw top container and shake.

Health benefits of this recipe.

Parsley is high in vitamin C. Helps regulate the adrenal glands. Helps the kidneys.

Radish Salad

Ingredients

6 radishes, sliced
2 carrots grated
1 small cucumber, chopped
2 stalks of celery, chopped
1 bunch baby spinach, tear into bite-sized pieces
white pepper, ground

Method

Toss together and place in a serving bowl.
Top with salad dressing.

Dressing

1/2 cup extra virgin olive oil
1/4 cup white wine vinegar
1 tbsp liquid honey
1/4 tsp Dijon mustard
1 tsp freshly chopped basil or parsley
black pepper, ground

Method

Place all dressing ingredients in a screw top container and shake.

Marcia's Tomato Salad

Ingredients

1kg of assorted tomatoes: cherry, Italian,
yellow, beefsteak
1/2 small jar sundried tomatoes, sliced
1 bunch of basil
black pepper, freshly ground

Method

Wash tomatoes and chop into chunks, wedges,
halves, depending on the tomato variety.
Place in a serving bowl. Add basil leaves
without stalks.
Slice sundried tomatoes and add to the bowl.
Toss gently.
Dress with sundried dressing before serving.

Health benefits of this recipe.

*Tomatoes benefit the kidneys and are high in vitamin C,
zinc, potassium, iron, magnesium and B vitamins.*

Sundried Tomato Dressing

Ingredients

6 tbsp extra virgin olive oil

2 tbsp sundried tomato oil

4 tbsp balsamic or white wine vinegar

1 clove garlic, crushed

black pepper, coarsely ground

Method

Place all ingredients in a screw top jar and shake. Toss gently through the tomatoes and basil.

Broccoli and Carrot Salad

Ingredients

1/2 cup broccoli, chopped

1/2 cup cauliflower, chopped

1 grated carrot

2 tbsp raisins

2 tbsp toasted sunflower seeds or pine nuts

Method

Place in a serving bowl and top with seeds and dressing. Toss.

Dressing

6 tbsp extra virgin olive oil

3 tbsp of lemon juice

black pepper, coarsely ground

Method

Place all ingredients in a screw top jar and shake. Toss gently through the salad.

Variations

You can blanch the cauliflower and broccoli first in boiling water 3 minutes. Take off the heat. Pour into sieve. Run under cold water to crisp. Drain and place in a serving bowl.

Warm Bean Salad

Ingredients

500g green beans
2 tsp olive oil
2 cloves garlic
3 tomatoes, chopped

Method

Blanch green beans in boiling water then rinse under cold water and drain.
Heat oil in a pan. Add garlic and chopped tomatoes. Stir fry together lightly and pour warm bean salad into a serving dish.

Grilled Pepper Salad

Ingredients

4 red bell peppers

4 yellow bell peppers

olive oil

pepper

6 fresh basil leaves

Method

Heat oven to 200 degrees C. Place pepper on a baking tray and roast, turning twice until the skins turn brown. Take out of oven and seal in a food-safe plastic bag. Leave for 20 minutes. Then peel the skin and cut in half and remove the seeds. Save the juice. Add a little olive oil to the juice and freshly ground black pepper. Slice peppers into thin strips. Pour juices over as a dressing. Top with shredded fresh basil. Serve at room temperature.

Marinated Mushroom Salad

Ingredients

1 punnet of raw button mushrooms, washed and sliced

Dressing

1/2 tsp fresh marjoram or oregano, chopped
cracked pepper

Method

Place mushrooms in a bowl. Add cracked pepper and chopped herbs.
Add dressing, toss. Refrigerate 30 minutes before serving.

Dressing

6 tbsp avocado or extra virgin olive oil

3 tbsp wine or champagne vinegar

Health benefits of this recipe.

Mushrooms are high in B vitamins, vitamin C and potassium. Parsley helps kidney function and is high in Vitamins C, E and A.

MARINADES AND SALSAS

All Seasons Marinade

Ingredients

1 cup olive

1/2 cup lemon juice

1 tbsp grated lemon zest, finely shredded

1/2 tsp cracked black pepper

2 tsp fresh herbs such as oregano, basil

Method

Mix all ingredients together in a bowl. Ideal marinade for chicken, meat and fish.

Health benefits of this recipe.
Lemons are high in vitamin C.

Cranberry and Balsamic Relish

Ingredients

1 red onion cut in wedges

1/2 cup balsamic vinegar

1 cup raw sugar

250g frozen cranberries

1 tsp crushed juniper berries

1/2 tsp ground allspice

Method

Bring all ingredients to a boil. Cook for 5 minutes covered. Then cook for 15 minutes uncovered, stirring frequently. Cool and pack into sterilized jars and store in the fridge. Perfect for cold meats and sandwiches.

Health benefits of this recipe.

Cranberries are good for the kidneys. High in vitamin C. Allspice is a healing spice with anti-inflammatory and antioxidant qualities. Juniper berries contain calcium, vitamin C, vitamin E and vitamin A.

Red Onion Jam

Ingredients

5 red onions, sliced thinly
1 1/2 cups brown sugar
2 tbsp olive oil
1/2 cup balsamic vinegar
black pepper, ground

Method

Heat oil in pan. Add sliced onions and cook carefully until transparent and soft. Add brown sugar stirring all the time over low heat until the onions become caramelized. Pour on balsamic and continue to cook stirring until the onion jam is slightly thick and aromatic. Grind over black pepper. Pour into clean jars or containers and seal. Store in fridge.

Health benefits of this recipe.

Red onions act as a healthy blood tonic and are high in potassium and zinc.

Winter Store Cupboard Relish

Ingredients

1 tbsp olive oil

1 cup red capsicum, chopped finely

1/2 sun-dried tomatoes

1 cup tinned no-salt tomatoes

1/4 cup balsamic vinegar

1/4 cup white wine vinegar - low acidity

1/2 cup raw sugar

pinch of allspice or cinnamon

1 tbsp of capers optional (soak in milk, then rinse and drain)

Method

Place all ingredients except capers in a saucepan. Cook on medium heat until reduced. About 20 minutes. Stir often. Add capers. Cook 5 minutes. Cool. Store in the fridge.

Health benefits of this recipe.
Red capsicum contains high levels of beta-carotene and vitamin C.

Creative Salsa Sauce

Ingredients

mango, peeled and chopped

melon

(watermelon, cantaloupe, honeydew) chopped

fresh tomato, chopped

fresh coriander, chopped

black pepper

olive oil,

chili green or red, (optional) seeds removed,

sliced thinly, julienne style

Method

Mix fruit and tomatoes together. Drizzle with olive oil. Grind black pepper over.

Health benefits of this recipe.

Mango contain beta-carotene so they are one of the highest antioxidant fruits. They also contain vitamin E and vitamin C and minerals such as potassium, zinc and magnesium. Honeydew melons contain high levels of vitamin C, beta-carotene and potassium. Cantaloupe melons are high in fiber, folate and vitamin C.

Tomato Salsa

Ingredients

1/2 cup of tinned tomatoes, chopped

1 tsp sweet chili sauce

1 tsp brown sugar

black pepper to taste

red or white onion, diced

fresh coriander, chopped

fresh coriander leaves

Method

Mix all ingredients together gently.
Place in a bowl and garnish with coriander leaves.

Health benefits of this recipe.
Coriander contains vitamins C, A, E and B's as well as minerals such as potassium and zinc.

Nectarine Salsa

Ingredients

two oranges, juice and grated rind

1 tbsp coriander, finely chopped

1/2 tsp fresh ginger, grated

1 small cinnamon stick

1 tsp honey

1/4 tsp ground cumin

40g raisins

4 nectarines cut in large chunks

Method

Combine orange juice, ginger, honey, cinnamon stick and cumin in a small saucepan.
Bring to the boil and simmer on low heat for two minutes. Add raisins and cool. Stir in nectarines, coriander and mix well. Store in jars in the fridge.

Health benefits of this recipe.
Nectarines have powerful antioxidants because they contain high levels of vitamin C, beta-carotene and potassium. Raisins improve circulation and are good for tissues and glands in the body.

Toulouse French Dressing

Ingredients

3 tbsp wine vinegar
or 3 tbsp fresh lemon juice
or 3 tbsp balsamic vinegar
6 tbsp extra virgin olive oil
ground black pepper
1 clove of garlic

Method

Cut the garlic and rub the clove around the inside of the salad bowl. Place all ingredients in a screw top container and shake. Pour over salad immediately before serving.

Variation

Add 1 tsp grainy mustard
Add 1 tsp Dijon mustard
Add chopped herbs
Add paprika
Add fresh basil, chopped
Add lots of garlic!

Plum Vinaigrette

Ingredients

2 tsp brown sugar

2 tsp French grainy mustard

6 tbsp olive oil

3 tbsp red wine vinegar

2 tbsp plum jam

Method

Mix all ingredients together. Serve as a dressing for roasted vegetables and salads of chicken and beef.

Corn and Pepper Relish

Ingredients

300g tin of diced no-salt tomatoes
2 red peppers, diced
3 cloves garlic
1 tbsp fresh oregano, chopped
I can whole kernel corn (no-sat) drained or 1
cup of fresh corn cooked and cut off the cob
olive oil

Method

Heat garlic gently in a frying pan. Add oregano
leaves, tomatoes, diced red peppers. Cook until
soft and aromatic. Add corn. Store in jars in the
fridge.

Health benefits of this recipe.
Corn is high in potassium.

VEGETABLES

Garlic Beans

Ingredients

fresh green beans, preferably ling snake beans
3 tbsp olive oil
3 cloves garlic, sliced
2 tsp fresh ginger, grated
black pepper

Method

Cut tops and tails off the beans. Cut beans in half. Blanch beans - place in boiling water for 1 minute and rinse with cold water. Drain.
Fry garlic in oil and ginger. Add beans and pepper. Stir fry 3 minutes.
Serve hot.

Health benefits of this recipe.
Green beans are high in fiber, protein, and vitamin B's.

Roasted Rosemary Potatoes

Ingredients

5 potatoes, washed, peeled and cubed

2 tbsp olive oil

fresh rosemary

4 cloves of garlic

black pepper

Method

Heat oven to 190 degrees C. Dry potatoes on kitchen paper. Place in roasting tray. Toss with olive oil and pepper. Grind black pepper. Place sprigs of fresh rosemary and garlic cloves in the tray. Bake for 30 minutes until golden.

Health benefits of this recipe.
Rosemary is a powerful antioxidant and it stimulates the circulation. Contains minerals such as magnesium, zinc, potassium and vitamins C,B's, A, E.

Eggplant Caponata

Ingredients

olive oil

2 eggplants (650g) cut into 3 pieces

2 sticks of celery, chopped

1 red onion, chopped

2 cloves of garlic, chopped

2 cups of Italian tomato sauce

1/2 cup red wine vinegar

3 tbsp chopped fresh basil

1 tsp sugar

Method

Heat oil. Cook eggplants in small batches on medium heat until browned. Drain on kitchen paper. Heat 1/4 cup of oil and cook celery and onion until transparent but not brown. Cook over low heat until soft. Add garlic, tomato sauce. Simmer for 10 minutes uncovered. Add the rest of the ingredients. Simmer for 10 minutes then add eggplant. Heat through. Serve with roast lamb cutlets with rosemary and mashed potato.

Health benefits of this recipe.
High in vitamin C, vitamin E and B vitamins.

Roasted Asparagus with Roasted Red Pepper Sauce

Ingredients

1 kg whole asparagus, stalks peeled with
potato peeler
garlic, finely crushed
olive oil
black pepper

Method

Heat oven to 200 degrees C. Paint baking tray
with olive oil. Sprinkle with garlic and course
black pepper. Spread the asparagus over the
bottom of the dish. Roast until the asparagus is
al dente. Do not over cook. Serve hot or warm
with the following sauce.

Roasted Red Pepper Puree

Ingredients

6 red capsicums (bell peppers), roasted, de-seeded and peeled
1 1/2 cups of roasted (unsalted) cashew nuts
2 cloves garlic
1 cup olive oil
1 tsp sugar
black pepper
balsamic vinegar

Method

Put all ingredients for the puree except the oil, vinegar and pepper into a food processor or blender. Puree. Add the oil very slowly as you blend to make a puree consistency. Taste and season. Serve with roasted asparagus.

Variation

Serve roasted red pepper puree with grilled fish or grilled chicken.

Health benefits of this recipe.

Asparagus assists the kidneys and eliminates toxins from the liver. Boosts the immune system with vitamin A, vitamin C and selenium, folate, vitamin B's.

Roasted Vegetables with Rosemary

Ingredients

aubergine

courgettes

red, yellow bell peppers (capsicum)

pumpkin

leeks

red onions

large mushrooms

garlic

2 tbsp balsamic vinegar

2 tsp of ground cumin

or leaves of fresh rosemary

Method

Wash and slice your selection of vegetables. Place in a roasting tin. Drizzle with olive oil and your choice of rosemary or cumin. Heat oven to 190 degrees C. Roast vegetables until golden and tender. When you take the tray from the oven drizzle with balsamic and extra virgin olive oil if desired.
Serve warm or cold.

Variation

Add one cup of cooked couscous and five tbsp raisins and 2 tbsp toasted pine nuts or pistachios to the cumin recipe.

Health benefits of this recipe.

Courgettes contain minerals such as iron, calcium, zinc, potassium, magnesium and vitamins C, B's as well as folate and fiber.

Provincial Ratatouille

Ingredients

2 red onions, chopped into chunks

2 green bell peppers, de-seeded and sliced

2 aubergine (eggplant) sliced into chunks

4 courgettes, sliced into chunks

750g Italian tomatoes, skinned and sliced

4 cloves garlic, peeled and finely chopped

2 tbsp chopped fresh basil leaves

olive oil for frying

Method

Fry garlic and onions in oil until they become transparent and soft. Add eggplant and courgettes until vegetables are cooked. Add tomatoes, basil and pepper and cook on low heat for 15 more minutes stirring constantly to prevent sticking. Add a little water if needed.

Variation

Serve hot or cold. As an appetizer with warm French bread, a main vegetable dish or a side dish to accompany meat.

124

Lavento Vegetable Frittata

Ingredients

2 potatoes, cut in small cubes and parboiled

1 clove garlic, crushed

1 red pepper, chopped

4 brown shallots or 1 onion, finely chopped

fresh basil leaves

oregano

3-4 eggs, beaten

olive oil

Method

Heat oil in a fry pan and add garlic and onions. Cook until transparent. Add potatoes and any other vegetables you like or have leftover. Cook for ten minutes on low heat. Flatten the vegetables to cover the base of the pan. Pour eggs over and top with basil leaves and a grind of black pepper. Cook until the bottom of the frittata is golden. Place under a grill to brown the top. Take care not to burn the base or the top. Cool slightly and tip upside down onto a serving plate. Serve in wedges with salad and salsa. Serve warm or cold.

Variation

This is a creative recipe and a great way of incorporating healthy vegetables or using up leftovers. Optional vegetables of your choice: broccoli, pumpkin, aubergine, mushrooms, corn, partly cooked and chopped into cubes.

MAIN COURSES

PASTA

Bruno's Spaghetti and Meatballs

Ingredients

250g minced beef

250g minced veal or pork

4 slices of day-old bread soaked in water and
squeezed dry

1 onion, grated

1 clove garlic, minced

2 tbsp minced fresh parley

1 tsp dried oregano
1/2 tsp freshly ground black pepper
2 eggs lightly beaten
olive oil
spaghetti

Method

Mix beef and veal. Tear bread into pieces
and add. Add onion, garlic, parsley, oregano
and pepper. Mix together. Add eggs and mix.
Shape into meatballs. Bake in a preheated
190 degrees C oven for 25 minutes. Or fry in a
pan over medium heat until brown and cooked
through. About 10 minutes.
To serve, cook spaghetti, drain and toss with
tomato pasta sauce in a large bowl. Serve
meatballs on top. Serves 6

Bruno's Spaghetti Arabiatta

Ingredients

3 tins Italian tomatoes, seeded and drained

1/4 cup olive oil

2 cloves garlic

1 tsp sugar

1 red chili, de-seeded (optional)

4 cups cooked pasta

2 tbsp fresh basil, ripped

black pepper, freshly ground

Method

Heat oil in a pan. Add garlic. Fry 30 seconds.
Add tomatoes, chili and sugar. Stir one minute
crushing the tomatoes. Pour over pasta. Add
basil, ground black pepper and add a drizzle of
extra virgin olive oil.
Serves 6-8

Variation

Add chicken, beef, seafood or capers to the
pan and cook with the garlic before adding
tomatoes.

Health benefits of this recipe.
Tomatoes assist kidney function. Tomatoes are high in

Lycopene, a phytochemical that helps the body resist infection. Cooking the tomatoes releases the Lycopene so tomato products such as pasta sauces, tomato sauce are good sources.

Bruno's Spaghetti Bolognaise

Ingredients

1 cup white button mushrooms, sliced

1 kg minced beef

2 large onions

2 tbsp unsalted butter

2 tbsp olive oil

4 cups canned low salt tomatoes

(or stew your own and remove the skins)

1 small can of no-salt/low salt tomato paste

1 tsp fresh oregano, chopped

2 tbsp fresh basil, chopped

black pepper, ground

Method

Cook onions in butter. Add beef, mushrooms
and brown. Add other ingredients. Simmer
uncovered, stirring occasionally for two hours.
Add water as necessary.
Season with pepper and freshly shredded basil
leaves. Serve on your choice of spaghetti or
pasta. Serves 6-8

Variation

Use leftover sauce to make a filling for an omelette. Add a can of rinsed and drained red kidney beans, 1 tsp ground cumin. Heat for ten minutes and fill taco shells. Top with avocado slices, shredded lettuce, freshly chopped tomatoes and a low salt tomato sauce.

Health benefits of this recipe.
Mushrooms contain protein, C, E and B vitamins, minerals such as selenium, zinc and potassium.

SEAFOOD

Big House Grilled Prawns

Ingredients

500-1kg fresh prawns, shelled and de-veined
thin bamboo skewers

Marinade

3/4 cup olive oil
1/4 cup lime zest
2 tsp thyme leaves
3 cloves garlic crushed
cracked black pepper

Method

Mix marinade ingredients. Thread prawns on
skewers. Pour marinade over. Marinate 30
minutes, turning occasionally before grilling.

Health benefits of this recipe.
Thyme has antioxidant and anti-inflammatory proper-
ties. Prawns are high in calcium, magnesium, potassi-
um, zinc.

Antonio's Steamed Mussels

Ingredients

1 1/2 cups white wine

2 kg live mussels in shells, cleaned

2 tsp olive oil

1 red chili deseeded (optional)

2 tbsp lemon zest, shredded

2 cloves garlic

1/4 cup lemon juice

1/2 cup white wine extra

cracked black pepper

cooked spaghetti to serve

chopped parsley to serve

Method

Bring wine to boil. Add mussels. Steam covered for 4 minutes. Drain. Remove one top shell on each mussel. Set aside. In a clean pan, heat the oil. Add leek, chili, lemon zest and garlic. Cook for 5-10 minutes. Take care not to burn. Add mussels, lemon juice, extra wine and pepper. Cook 2 minutes. Serve on top of spaghetti with tomato mussel sauce and parsley.

Health benefits of this recipe.
Mussels have known anti-inflammatory properties and are high in protein and zinc.

Pacific Island Prawn Curry

Ingredients

800g prawns, peeled and de-veined

1/2 cup vegetable oil

1 onion, chopped

3 cloves garlic, finely chopped

1 1/2 tsp turmeric

1 mild green chili de-seeded and finely chopped (optional)

3 tsp ground cumin

2 tsp fresh minced ginger root

1/2 tsp fenugreek, whole

1/2 tsp ground cinnamon

1/2 tsp sugar

1 tin coconut milk

2 tbsp fresh coriander for garnish

1 tsp garam marsala for garnish

Method

Heat oil in pan. Add onions, garlic and chili and fry until transparent. Take care not to burn. Add sugar and all the dry spices. Stir and fry for 4 minutes more. Don't burn. Add coconut cream and simmer on low until it thickens slightly.

Brown the prawns in another pan. Add the
coconut mixture to them. Simmer until cooked.
Garnish with a sprinkle of garam masala
powder and fresh coriander leaves. Serve with
steamed rice.

Variation

Substitute your favorite seafood. Crayfish,
scallops, crab, snapper, any white fish or
shellfish in place of the prawns.

Health benefits of this recipe.

*Turmeric helps blood flow, stimulates the liver and has
anti-inflammatory properties. Cinnamon benefits the
heart, liver and kidneys. Fenugreek contains antioxidants and helps the function of the liver and pancreas.*

Marinated Calamari

Ingredients

500g small squid

1 tbsp olive oil

1 tbsp lemon zest

2 tbsp lemon juice

2 tbsp thyme leaves

black pepper, cracked

Method

Cut squid into 4 strips. Mix all marinade
ingredients and pour over squid. Marinate for 1
hour. Cook on hot grill for 3-4 minutes.

Health benefits of this recipe.
*Squid are low-fat salt-water fish that are high in protein,
calcium and iodine.*

Mum's Fish Cakes

Ingredients
2 large potatoes
white pepper, ground
2 teaspoons of capers, soaked in milk then
rinsed and drained (optional)
1 cup of cooked fish (fresh white fish or low salt
tinned tuna or salmon)
flour for dipping
1 egg beaten
1 cup breadcrumbs, toasted white
tomato sauce, low salt

Method
Boil the potatoes in water until soft, drain and
mash. Add a grind of white pepper or a few
drained green peppercorns or washed capers.
Mix fish and potatoes together. Form into
cakes. Place in fridge for 30 minutes. Dip in
flour and egg and then crumbs and place each
cake on baking paper. Bake in a 190 degrees
C until crispy and golden. Serve with tomato
sauce or salsa and a salad.

Health benefits of this recipe.
Potatoes are rich in potassium and the B vitamins.

Atlantic Salmon with Spices

Ingredients

1 large piece of fresh salmon

1 tbsp coriander seeds

1 tsp turmeric powder

1 tbsp cumin seeds

black pepper, coarsely ground

Method

Wash the salmon and pat dry with kitchen paper. Cut the salmon into steaks with a sharp knife, keeping the skin on. Crush coriander seeds, cumin seeds and add turmeric powder and ground black pepper. Rub the spices onto the salmon skin. Cook gently on a grill or in a grill pan. Note that the oil in the fish will be enough to make the skin crispy. Serve on a bed of mashed potatoes. Add a dash of Japanese wasabi paste to the potato for extra flavor.

Health benefits of this recipe.
Salmon is rich in omega-3 essential fatty acids. Fish oils are well-known to lower cholesterol, improve circulation and protect the heart as well as anti-inflammatory properties. Cumin has antioxidant properties and is high in calcium, iron, potassium, zinc, magnesium, vitamin C.

Fish with Spicy Garlic Marinade

Ingredients

2 tbsp extra-virgin olive oil

2 tbsp wine vinegar

3 garlic cloves

1/2 tsp ground cumin

1/2 tsp dried oregano

2 tsp sweet paprika

black pepper

500 - 1kg fish cut in medium size pieces

olive oil

1 cup unbleached plain flour

Method

Mix vinegar, olive oil, garlic, cumin, paprika, oregano and black pepper. Add fish and mix. Marinate for 4 hours or up to 3 days. Remove fish from marinade. Place each piece of fish in flour and coat well. Heat 4 tablespoons of olive oil in a pan or a wok. Cook fish 2-3 minutes until golden brown. Serve on a bed of mashed pumpkin with lemon or lime wedges.

Health benefits of this recipe.
Fish is high in EPA's. Every cell and organ in the body needs essential fatty acids EPA's every day.

POULTRY

Chicken Burger

Ingredients

1kg chicken breasts, minced
1 egg
1/4 - 1/2 cup fresh breadcrumbs to bind
1 - 2 tsp green peppercorns
ground white pepper

Method

Place all ingredients in a bowl and mix well.
Shape into burgers and leave in the fridge
30 minutes to 1 hour before baking on an
oiled tray in a 180 degrees C oven for 20 -
30 minutes until cooked through. Serve in a
hamburger bun with cranberry sauce or relish
with leafy greens.

Turkey Burger

Ingredients

1kg turkey breast, minced

1 egg

1/4 - 1/2 cup fresh breadcrumbs to bind

1 apple, grated, juice squeezed out

1 tsp chopped sage leaves

ground white pepper

Method

Place all ingredients in a bowl and mix well. shape into burgers and leave in the fridge 30 minutes to 1 hour before baking on an oiled tray in a 180 degrees C oven for 20 - 30 minutes until cooked through. Serve in a hamburger bun with cranberry sauce or relish with leafy greens.

Health benefits of this recipe.
Turkey is high in protein and contains essential amino acid. Turkey is known to help insomnia.

Deli Style Chicken Breasts

Ingredients

1 kg whole chicken breasts, skinless

olive oil

black pepper

Filling choices

cranberry sauce

pesto made with basil and pinenuts

sundried tomato pesto

soft figs

dried apricots, soaked 30 minutes

Method

Place chicken breasts on chopping board
and cover with kitchen wrap. Take a rolling
pin or meat mallet and pound the pieces until
they become flat and thin. Wipe each piece
generously with your choice of filling and roll up
with the filling inside. You will have a sausage
like shape. Brush each one with oil. Place in
a heated oven 180 degrees C and bake until
golden and cooked. Serve sliced on a serving
plate with salad and roasted vegetables. Or use
in sandwiches, pita bread or with salad.

Ginger Chicken Curry

Ingredients

500g - 1kg meat for curry: use chicken breast, pork, fish, seafood, diced or in chunks
1 cardamom pod
1 bay leaf
freshly ground black pepper
1/4 tsp to 1/2 tsp of the following spices
cumin seeds
grated nutmeg
chopped mint
coriander seeds
turmeric
fennel seeds
fresh ginger root
2 tins chopped Italian tomatoes in juice, no-salt
2 tbsp tomato paste
1 onion, chopped
2 garlic cloves
2 tbsp olive oil
coriander leaves for garnish

Method

Grind spices together in a clean coffee grinder or a mortar and pestle. Fry onions and garlic in a little oil until transparent and soft. Do not brown. Add tomatoes and tomato paste. Add aromatic seeds and spices. Cook diced chicken, or pork, or fish/seafood in a little olive oil until lightly brown. Add to the tomato spice mix and simmer over low heat until the meat is cooked through. Serve with rice and coriander leaves.

Serves 4-6 people

Variation

Vary the spices to suit your taste buds. You can use any fish or meat. Vary the meat to change the flavor.

Health benefits of this recipe.

Cardamom contains vitamin B's, and C as well as minerals such as zinc and potassium and iron. Nutmeg helps restore the body's fluid metabolism. Fennel helps kidney function.

Cajun Barbecued Chicken

Ingredients

1 kg fresh chicken pieces

1/4 cup unsalted butter

2 garlic cloves, minced

1 tsp paprika, sweet and smoky kind

1 tsp dry mustard powder

1/2 tsp black pepper, ground

1/2 tsp white pepper, ground

1/2 tsp oregano

1/2 tsp thyme

Method

Combine butter with all the seasonings. Barbecue chicken and ten minutes before the chicken is ready, brush with the seasoned butter. Baste with the seasoned butter this will make the chicken blackened and smoky, with tender moist meat under the blackened skin in true Cajun style.

Health benefits of this recipe.
Paprika has anti-inflammatory properties and helps to boost the immune system. High in Vitamin A, C, B's and vitamin E.

Chicken Jambalaya

Ingredients

2 cups cooked chicken

1 cup onion, chopped

1 cup green capsicum, chopped

1 tbsp garlic, cut in fine slivers

3 cups Italian tomatoes, peeled, de-seeded and chopped

1 cup unsalted chicken stock (broth)

1 cup tomato juice, no-salt

1/2 tsp dried thyme

1 bay leaf

1/2 tsp ground pepper

3/4 cup white rice (risotto style rice)

250g scallops (optional)

500 - 1kg prawns or jumbo shrimp

1/2 cup parsley, chopped

olive oil

Method

Cook onions, green capsicum and garlic until aromatic. Add tomatoes, chicken stock, thyme, bay leaf. Simmer gently for ten minutes uncovered. Heat oven to 180 degrees C. Stir

in rice. Simmer 15 minutes. Add chicken,
scallops, shrimp and chicken. Cover and bake
30 minutes stirring twice.

Health benefits of this recipe.

Parsley is beneficial for the kidneys. Flat leaf parsley or Italian parsley has more nutrients than English parsley, but both are high in vitamin C, vitamin E, vitamin A. Rice is a good source of protein, complex carbohydrates and fiber and contains essential amino acids such as lysine.

Grilled Thai Chicken Salad

Ingredients

2 raw chicken breast fillets, sliced

3 tbsp fresh lime juice

1 tsp brown palm sugar grated

1 cup cooked rice vermicelli

mint leaves

spring onion

100g salad leaves

1 Lebanese cucumber, skin on, sliced

1/4 cup coriander

roasted peanuts without salt, chopped

Method

Place chicken, lime, sugar and toss. Heat fry
pan. Add chicken and marinade. Cover and
cook 4 minutes or until cooked. Take off heat.
Toss mint, spring onions and rice vermicelli
with chicken. Place on the salad greens and
top with cucumber and coriander leaves and
roasted peanuts.

Health benefits of this recipe.
*Cucumber helps with nerves and helps the body's fluid
balance. The skin contains high quantities of vitamin A.
Salad greens - a good source of fiber and nutrients*

40 Cloves of Garlic Roast Chicken

Ingredients

1.7 - 2kg whole chicken

1 tablespoon extra virgin olive oil

1 tsp rosemary

1 tsp thyme

1 bay leaf

1 onion, cut in half

1 lemon, cut in half

2 tsp freshly ground black pepper

20 - 40 garlic cloves, peeled

1 cup no-salt chicken stock or broth

1 cup dry white wine

French bread baguette

3 tbsp fresh flat-leaf parsley, chopped

Method

Rinse and dry chicken. Place in a roasting dish. Add lemon and herbs into the body cavity. Brush chicken with olive oil and grind over black pepper. Add chicken stock to the pan and add the garlic cloves. Roast in a preheated oven at 190-200 degrees C for an hour or until the chicken is cooked and a skewer inside the leg shows clear juices and not pink. Place on a serving dish surrounded by garlic. Serve with warm, crusty French bread and mash the cooked garlic cloves onto the bread for a sweet nutty garlic taste. Serve with a leafy green salad or steamed asparagus and French dressing.

Health benefits of this recipe.

Garlic enhances the immune system, treats infection and helps with blood circulation and fatigue. Bay leaf aids relaxation and helps relieve stress.

South Seas Coconut Curry

Ingredients

500 - 1kg meat or fish (chicken, pork, fish, shellfish)

2 stalks lemongrass, chopped (use tender yellow part, but not the leaves)

1 large bunch fresh coriander, chopped (use roots, stalks and leaves)

1 tbsp fresh ginger root, peeled, and finely chopped

1 bay leaf, crumbled

1 onion, chopped

3 tsp olive oil

2 cloves garlic, finely chopped

1 can coconut milk

2 spring onions, julienne for garnish

coriander leaves for garnish

Method

Mix herbs with coconut milk and set aside. Fry onion and garlic in a little oil, on medium heat, stirring until soft and transparent. Take care not to burn. Add your choice of meat or fish chopped into small chunks. Use any of the following, chicken, pork, fish or shellfish. Brown with the onions a little, and then add the coconut mixture and cook gently on a low heat until the meat is cooked through, stirring occasionally. Serve with rice and garnish with spring onions and fresh coriander leaves. Serves 4 - 8 people

Health benefits of this recipe.
Coconut is known as one of the world's super foods.

BEEF

Fillet of Beef with Salsa Verde

Ingredients

1 whole eye fillet about 1kg

7 tbsp extra virgin olive oil

1 1/2 large bunches Italian parsley

2 tbsp capers (optional) soaked in milk, rinsed and drained

1 1/2 tbsp onions, chopped

2 cloves garlic, chopped

1/2 zest of one lemon

1 tbsp white wine vinegar

2 potatoes, peeled and boiled

pepper to taste

Method

Preheat oven to 225 degrees C. Place fillet in the oven with 2 tsp of oil. Cook 15 minutes. Turn and cook another 15 minutes for rare. Meanwhile make the sauce. Combine all ingredients except remaining oil into a food processor. Add the oil in slowly to make the consistency of a mayonnaise. Let meat rest for 10 minutes after it is cooked. Spoon the green salsa around the edge of the serving plate. Carve the meat into 1 cm thick slices and place on the serving platter.

Health benefits of this recipe.

Red meat is high in iron, calcium, amino acids and minerals.

Cajun Meat Loaf

Ingredients

1 tbsp oil

2 onions, chopped

4 garlic cloves

2 tbsp minced sun-dried tomatoes

1/2 cup tomato paste

1 tsp cumin powder

1 kg beef mince

1/2 cup soft white breadcrumbs

1/2 cup skim milk

Method

Heat oven to 180 degrees C. Heat oil. Sauté onions and garlic until soft. Mix ingredients and add beef and breadcrumbs. Bake in a loaf tin for 1 - 1 1/2 hours till cooked Let rest 10 minutes before cutting. Serve with fresh tomato salsa or relish.

Fresh Tomato Salsa

Ingredients

1 1/2 cups tomatoes, chopped

1/2 cup onion, chopped

1/2 cup fresh cilantro, chopped

1 tsp sugar

2 tbsp vinegar

Method

Place all ingredients in a bowl and stir. Keep in jars in the fridge.

Beef Kebabs

Ingredients

1 kg of beef (sirloin, eye fillet or rump)
or 1 kg boned lamb, remove fat

Marinade

125 ml olive or safflower oil
2 onions finely chopped
2 tbsp of fresh mint, marjoram or oregano
finely chopped
ground black pepper
bamboo skewers soaked in water
red or yellow capsicum
baby onions
garlic cloves
cherry tomatoes or tomatoes in wedges
button mushrooms

Method

Mix marinade together. Cut meat into 2.5
cm cubes and toss in the marinade mix.
Refrigerate for at least one hour covered. Place
cubes of meat in bamboo skewers soaked
in water. Place marinated meat on skewers
alternating with vegetables. Grill or barbecue.

Variation

Moroccan marinade: Add 1-2 tsp cumin, 1 tsp paprika and 3 cloves of crushed garlic and the juice of one lemon to the marinade. When cooked serves garnished with lemon wedges, parsley and mint leaves.

Italian marinade: Use veal, lamb, chicken or pork. Omit Moroccan spices. Add 2 cloves crushed garlic, 2 tbsp chopped basil leaves, 1 tsp dried oregano and 1 crushed bay leaf added to the marinade. When cooked serve garnished with fresh basil leaves and tomato wedges.

Health benefits of this recipe.

Marjoram is high in magnesium, zinc, potassium, vitamin C and Vitamin A. Safflower oil contains vitamin E to help boost the immune system.

LAMB

Lamb Shanks

Ingredients

6 lamb shanks trimmed of fat

1/4 cup olive oil

2 onions, finely sliced

3 carrots, thinly sliced

3 cloves garlic, peeled and minced

1 bay leaf, fresh or dried

4 sprigs fresh oregano

2 stalks celery, sliced thinly

1/2 cup fresh Italian parsley, minced

1 1/2 cup of red wine

black pepper, ground

2 heads of garlic unpeeled and separated into cloves

1 can of Italian tomatoes in juice

1 tbsp tomato paste

3 sprigs of fresh rosemary

14 mushrooms, small

Method

Heat oven to 190 degrees C. Heat oil in a pan
and brown lamb shanks. Remove shanks.
Reduce heat and add onions, garlic, carrots,
oregano, bay leaf, celery, tomatoes, tomato
paste, red wine, and parsley. Cook and thicken
for 5 to 10 minutes. Add the lamb shanks to
a baking dish and all the peeled garlic. Add
tomato mixture. Put rosemary on top. Cover
with lid or tin foil. Turn lamb shanks every 20
minutes. Uncover. Add mushrooms. Cook a
further 30 minutes uncovered until the lamb
is very tender. Remove any fat from the pan.
Serve hot with mashed potatoes.

Health benefits of this recipe.

*Celery helps regulate the nervous system and control
dizziness and headaches. Carrots are the best source
of beta-carotene which helps boost the immune system,
builds healthy tissue. Rosemary is a powerful anti-inflammatory and helps improve circulation.*

Lamb Florentine

Ingredients

2 kg lamb leg, boned

1 tsp garlic, crushed

2 tbsp chopped parsley

2 tbsp unsalted butter

black pepper

1 jar of apricot or plum fruit chutney

Method

Mix butter and herbs and garlic into a paste.
Slit the skin of lamb to make pockets and stuff
with herb paste. Rub the leg with 2 tbsp of olive
oil and black pepper. Coat the lamb leg with
a fruity apricot or plum chutney. Cook for one
hour at 190 degrees C or until tender and the
juices are clear when pierced with a skewer.
In the last 15 minutes pour 2 tbsp of red wine
vinegar over the lamb. Then coat with a mixture
of 3 tbsp soft white breadcrumbs and 2 tbsp
soft unsalted butter if you want a golden crust.

Health benefits of this recipe.
*Apricots benefit the nerve tissues and are high in vita-
min C and vitamin B's.*

Kashmiri Lamb

Ingredients

1 kg leg of lamb
1 tbsp of garam masala, cumin and ground cardamom
500g Greek yogurt
8 strands of saffron
2 tbsp ground pistachios
2 tbsp of liquid honey

Method

Make deep cuts in the lamb. Mix together the spices and rub them over the lamb. Mix yogurt with honey and chopped pistachios and rub them over the lamb. Drizzle the honey over the top. Marinate for two to three days. Heat oven to 170 degrees C and slow cook for 3-1/2 hours. Serve with rice. Serves 8.

Health benefits of this recipe.
Saffron is an antioxidant and helps improve circulation.

PORK

Roast Pork with Apple Stuffing

Ingredients

2.8 kg boneless pork loin
oil for rubbing

Stuffing

2 tbsp oil
2 onions
3 apples sliced
1/4 cup brown sugar
2 tbsp sage leaves chopped
4 cups fresh white breadcrumbs

Method

Heat oven to 220 degrees C. Fry onions
until soft. Add apples. Cook until soft and

golden. Remove from heat and add sage
and breadcrumbs. Make a pocket in the pork
between the skin and the meat. Stuff this
pocket with stuffing. Rub oil on the skin.
Bake 30 minutes. Reduce to 200 degrees C
and bake for another 45 - 50 minutes.
Serves 8 -12.

Health benefits of this recipe.
Antioxidant and contains calcium, magnesium, potassium and zinc as well as vitamins C, B's and A.

Pork and Apple Burgers

Ingredients

1 kg minced pork

1 green apple, grated, juice squeezed

1 tsp dried sage leaves chopped

1 onion finely chopped

white pepper, freshly ground

Method

Mix pork, onion and apples with sage. Shape into burgers. Bake in a 190 degrees C until cooked through. Serve in toasted burger buns topped with a slice of fresh pineapple, grated carrot or any of your favorite toppings.

Health benefits of this recipe.
Pork is high in B vitamins and protein.

DESSERTS

Baked Peaches with Maple Syrup

Ingredients

one peach per person
4 tbsp pure maple syrup
1 tbsp lime or lemon juice

Method

Heat oven to 180 degrees C. Cut the peaches in half and remove the stone. Place in a baking dish cut side up. Add 2 tbsp of water into the dish. Pour on maple syrup, lemon juice and grind white pepper over the peaches. Put lid on the baking dish or cover with foil. Cook till tender but not falling apart. Serve with whipped cream or yogurt.

Sticky Rice with Coconut

Ingredients

1 cup glutinous white rice, soaked 8 hours, and drained

1/4 cup jasmine rice, washed

800ml coconut milk (thin)

700 ml milk

1/2 cup grated palm sugar

1/2 desiccated coconut, toasted

fresh mangoes, sliced

Method

Place all ingredients in a large saucepan. Bring slowly to boil, stir and simmer. Stir occasionally until thick. Pour the mixture into a dish lined with plastic wrap. Cover and chill overnight. Turn out onto a plate. Serve with fresh mango.

Fruit Salad

Ingredients

1/2 cup dark palm sugar, grated

1/2 cup water

400 ml coconut cream

3 cups mixed tropical fruit

1 cup of crushed ice

Method

Make a palm sugar syrup by dissolving the grated palm sugar with water and bringing to the boil. Stir until dissolved. Cool and chill. Mix everything together in a chilled bowl and add the palm sugar syrup to taste.

Health benefits of this recipe.
Tropical fruits are a great source of vitamin C and potassium.

Amaretto Baked Peaches

Ingredients

4 peaches, halved and stoned
110g Italian amaretto biscuits, crushed
50g castor sugar
50g unsalted butter, softened
1 egg yolk

Method

Scoop out a little of the peach flesh. Mash together with biscuits, sugar, butter and egg yolk. Fill peach halves with mixture. Place peaches in a baking dish with 4 tbsp water in the bottom. Bake at 180 degrees C for 25 minutes until golden but still firm.

Variation

Use a mixture of ground almonds with a few teaspoons of unsalted butter and dark cane sugar and a drop of almond essence.

Health benefits of this recipe.
Peaches are high in vitamin C, potassium, zinc, magnesium, vitamin B's, vitamin E and vitamin K.

Baked Almond Apricots

Ingredients

1 kg apricots

125 g ground almonds

125 g caster sugar

1 tsp almond essence

1-2 tbsp unsalted butter

Method

Heat oven to 180 degrees C. Wash apricots, cut in half and remove the stone. Place in a lightly greased baking dish. Make an almond paste by mixing caster sugar and almonds together with almond essence and butter. Fill the halves with almond paste. Cover dish with foil and bake for 20 minutes until firm but cooked and the paste golden.

Health benefits of this recipe.
Almonds are known as a super nut because they are high in potassium, calcium, protein, magnesium and folic acid.

Snitterfield Summer Berry Pudding

Ingredients

1 loaf of fresh white bread cut into thin slices
unsalted butter
1 cup each of any of the following summer
berries: blueberries, strawberries, raspberries,
loganberries, blackberries, blackcurrants,
redcurrants,(fresh or frozen are fine)

Method

Place berries in a non-corrosive pan and add
a little clear honey or sugar to sweeten to
taste. Simmer gently just until the juice flows.
Cut crusts off the bread and butter one side.
Place bread slices butter side down and line a
pudding basin. Carefully spoon in the berries.
Pour the juice over the berries. Make a lid of
bread. Then place a plate on top and a weight
on top to press the pudding into shape. Place
the weighted pudding into the fridge for 1 day.
Turn out carefully by running a knife between
the bread and the bowl. Turn out and cut into
slices. Serve with a little light cream or vanilla
custard.

Health benefits of this recipe.

Blueberries are a powerful antioxidant. Strawberries are full of super nutrients. High in vitamin C and potassium. Blackcurrants and redcurrants are high in fiber and vitamin C and have antibacterial and anti-inflammatory properties.

Tahitian Vanilla Bean Custard

Ingredients

6 egg yolks

1/4 cup caster sugar

2 tbsp corn flour

1/3 cup milk

3 cups light cream

1tsp vanilla extract

I vanilla bean, split, scraped and seeds
reserved

Method

Place egg yolks in a bowl and beat together
with caster sugar. Mix milk with corn flour and
add cream and vanilla extract and vanilla bean
pulp and seeds. Add slowly to the egg mixture
and mix until all ingredients are combined.
Cook in a pan over boiling water until it
thickens. Take care not to boil the egg and
cream mixture. Stir constantly until it thickens.

Health benefits of this recipe.
Vanilla comes from seed pods of a special orchid plant.
Vanilla is rich in antioxidants.

Brioche with Berry Sauce

Ingredients

1 1/2 tsp dried yeast

150 ml warm milk

250g flour

4 eggs beaten

3 tbsp sugar

160g unsalted butter

zest of lemon, finely chopped

Method

Preheat oven to 170 degrees C. Dissolve yeast in warm water. Stir in flour, eggs and sugar. Beat well. Cover and let rise until double in bulk. Punch down. Add butter and lemon zest. Pour into a greased brioche tin. Cover and let dough rise again. Bake 20-25 minutes till a skewer comes out clean. Serve with warm berry sauce.

Berry Sauce

Ingredients

200g of fresh berries

juice of 1/2 an orange

1/4 cup of water

1/2 cup of raw sugar

Method

Put half the berries in a small pan with sugar
and orange juice and bring to the boil. Cool.
Stir in the rest of the berries. Cool completely.
Serve with warm brioche.

Health benefits of this recipe.
*Eggs contain vitamin B's, iron and zinc. Raspberries are
great for the kidneys and the blood.*

Eve's Baked Apples

Ingredients

4-6 apples (1 for each person)
1/4-1/2 cup ground almonds
6-8 tbsp of dried apricots or other dried
fruits (raisins, dates, cherries, blueberries,
cranberries, peaches)
3-6 tsp unsalted butter
2-4 tsp dark brown sugar
1/4 tsp cinnamon

Method

Preheat oven to 180 degrees C. Core apples
but leave the skin on. Mix ingredients together
into a paste. Fill each apple with the mixture.
Place apples upright in a baking dish. Add 1/4
cup of water to the bottom of the dish. Cover
with foil. Bake 180 degree C for 20-30 minutes
until apples are cooked but not falling apart.

Health benefits of this recipe.
*Dates are potassium rich and are high in vitamin B's
and C. Cherries are high in vitamin C.*

Honey Spiced Rice Pudding

Ingredients

75g short-grain white rice

1.5 liters milk

50g-75g sugar

3 tbsp honey

3 tbsp rose water or 1 tsp vanilla essence

2 tbsp pistachio nuts or almond, chopped finely

75g pistachio nuts, almonds or hazelnuts, toasted and finely chopped

Method

Place the rice in a pan of water, bring to the boil and boil for 5 minutes and drain. Bring the milk to the boil, add rice and simmer over a low heat, stirring to prevent sticking until the rice is creamy. Add the sugar and honey and rosewater or vanilla. Stir and simmer for 5 minutes over low heat. Serve in bowls with nuts sprinkled over the top. Serve either hot or cold. Serves 6.

Health benefits of this recipe.
Pistachio nuts are high in protein, calcium, iron, potassium, magnesium and zinc.

Far North Tropical Fruit salad

Ingredients

1 fresh papaya, deseeded and sliced
1 banana, sliced
1 small pineapple, chopped
1 mango, sliced
2 passion fruit, flesh scooped out
1 lime juiced or 1/4 cup pineapple juice
mint leaves for garnish
honey

Method

Place papaya, pineapple, passion fruit and mango in a bowl. Pour lime juice or pineapple juice over the fruit to prevent browning. Toss. Garnish with mint leaves. Serve with plain yogurt and a drizzle of honey.

Variation

Use orange juice, lemon juice or passion fruit juice to replace lime juice. Use any fruits in season.

Blueberry and Grape Fruit Salad

Ingredients

1 punnet of blueberries

1 red or green apple, skin on

1 peach or nectarine, sliced

1/2 cup green or red seedless grapes

1 small pineapple, chopped

1 banana

honey

1/2 packet slivered almonds, toasted

Method

Slice the banana, peach and apple into a bowl. Add grapes and pineapple. Toss and serve. Garnish with toasted slivered almonds. Serve with yogurt.

Health benefits of this recipe.
Grapes increase energy. They strengthen the kidneys and are high in vitamin C.

Mango Crumble

Ingredients

5 mango, peeled and sliced, pip removed

8 tbsp raw sugar

8 tbsp unbleached white flour or wholemeal

6 tbsp oats

1 tsp ground cinnamon

1/4 tsp ground nutmeg

4 tbsp unsalted butter

Method

Heat oven to 180 degrees C. Place mango in a baking dish. Mix the oats, flour, sugar and spices together and then add the butter. Crumble the butter through to make a soft topping. Sprinkle over the mangoes and bake until golden brown, 25-30 minutes.

Variation

Use 5 apples instead of mangoes. Use frozen berries such as blueberries. Use berries and apple combination.

Eve's Apple Crumble

Ingredients

5 cups of finely sliced apples

1 1/2 tsp ground cinnamon

1/2 cup maple syrup or liquid honey

1/4 cup unsalted butter

1/2 cup oats

1/2 cup unbleached flour

1/4 cup raisins

Method

Heat oven to 180 degrees C. Butter a baking dish. Mix cinnamon and raisins with apples and place in the dish. If apples are tart, add a little raw sugar to taste. Mix maple syrup of honey with butter. Add oats and mix. Spread over the apples and brush with a little melted butter. Bake 25-30 minutes until golden. Serve warm.

Variation

Substitute fresh or frozen berries or stone fruit, such as apricots for the apples.

DRINKS

Lemon Mint Refresher

Ingredients

1 liter of water
juice of 3 lemons or 3 limes
1/2 teaspoon of honey
mint leaves, chopped
6 ice cubes

Method

Place lemon or lime juice in a jug. Add honey and mint leaves. Add water. Stir. Add ice.

Variation

Blend in a blender with ice cubes to make a summer chiller.

Carrot and Ginger Drink

Ingredients

3 large carrots, washed and peeled, green tops
removed
2 tbsp fresh ginger root, washed and peeled
1/2 cup water
1 tsp honey

Method

Place all ingredients in a blender and blend
until smooth. Drink straight away.

Ginger Tea

Ingredients

1 piece of fresh ginger root (size of index finger), washed and peeled
water
1 tsp honey
lemon juice to taste

Method

Grate the fresh ginger root into a china teapot. Bring water to the boil and pour over the ginger. Seep the tea for five minutes. Strain. Serve with honey. If a little strong add more boiling water.

Variation

You can serve with ice and mint as a refreshing summer drink.

Lemon Honey Tea

Ingredients

1/2 - 1 lemon or lime, squeezed, pips removed
honey
boiling water

Method

Place lemon juice in a cup. Pour boiling over the lemon juice. Add honey to taste. Stir. Serve hot or cold in summer with ice and mint.

Cranberry and Apple Juice

Ingredients

1 medium to large apple, including skin, pips
except the stalk
1/2 cup of cranberries, fresh or frozen
water
honey to taste

Method

Place ingredients in a blender and blend until
smooth. Add honey and ice. Drink straight
away.

Health benefits of this recipe.
*Apple juice is high in minerals and is good for cleansing,
and detoxifying the body.*

Apple, Celery and Cucumber Juice

Ingredients

1 medium cucumber, skin on

2 green apples, skin and pips

2 stalks of celery

1 small bunch of parsley

water

mint leaves, washed

Method

Place cucumber, apples and parsley into a juicer. Juice. Add water and ice cubes and a few mint leaves to garnish.

Variation

Add mint leaves to the juicer. Add a small handful of watercress leaves as they help oxygenate the blood and contain concentrated nutrients so use sparingly in juices.

Health benefits of this recipe.
Cucumber and celery helps the body maintain the correct sodium and potassium balance.

Queen's Barley Water

Ingredients

1 cup pearl barley, washed

1 liter of boiling water

3 oranges, juiced

1 lemon, rind and juice

raw sugar to taste

Method

Place washed barley in a large saucepan and add boiling water. Simmer over low heat with lid on for 1 hour. Strain water from barley adding rind from lemon. Add sugar. Allow to cool then strain the lemon rind, remove. Add the juice of 3 oranges and 1 lemon. Stir and keep in the fridge. Allow to stand. Drink hot or cold.

Health benefits of this recipe.
Barley is potassium rich and contains important vitamins and minerals such as zinc, vitamin E, magnesium, calcium and protein.

SPICE TEAS

Allspice Tea

Seep 1-2 teaspoons of crushed allspice seeds
or powder in one cup of boiling water.
Leave for 20 minutes. Strain and serve.

Health benefits of this recipe.
Anti-inflammatory properties.

Anise Tea

Crush 1 tsp of anise seeds. Add to a teapot and
pour over boiling water. Seep for 10 minutes,
strain and drink.

Health benefits of this recipe.
High in vitamins C, A and E.

Bay Leaf Tea

Place 2 teaspoons of dried bay leaves in a teapot. Pour on one cup of boiling water. leave for 10 minutes. Strain.

Health benefits of this recipe.
Helps with relaxation and relieving stress.

Cardamom Tea

Crush 1 tsp of cardamom seeds or use 1tsp of powdered cardamom. Place in a pot and pour boiling water over. Leave 10 minutes. Strain before drinking.

Health benefits of this recipe.
An energy booster.

Fennel Tea

Crush 2 tsp of fennel seeds and add a cup of boiling water. Seep for ten minutes then strain and serve.

Health benefits of this recipe.
Fennel is good for treating symptoms of vertigo and nausea.

Marjoram Tea

Use 2 tsp of dried leaves per cup of boiling water. Infuse for 5 -10 minutes and serve.

Health benefits of this recipe.
Marjoram is used to prevent motion sickness and alleviate insomnia.

Mint Tea

Place 1/2 cup of fresh mint leaves on a chopping board. Sprinkle 2 tsp of raw sugar over the leaves then shred the mint with a sharp knife. Place in a jug and pour over 4 cups of water. Let stand for 15 minutes. Serve with lemon. Hot or cold.

Health benefits of this recipe.
Mint helps relieve nervous tension.

Oregano Tea

Place 1-2 tsp in a pot, add boiling water and infuse for ten minutes.

Health benefits of this recipe.
Oregano has been used for centuries to treat vomiting and is a powerful antioxidant.

Sage Tea

Place 1-2 tsp dried sage leaves in a pot. Add 1 cup of boiling water. Infuse for ten minutes. Strain and drink.

Health benefits of this recipe.
Sage has antioxidant properties.

Thyme Tea

Place 2 tsp of thyme in a teapot. Add a cup of boiling water. Infuse for ten minutes before drinking.

Health benefits of this recipe.
Thyme is a powerful antioxidant.

FAMILY FAVORITES

CAKES BREADS AND MUFFINS

Honey Bee Bread

Ingredients

1 packet of active dry yeast
1 1/2 cups lukewarm water
pinch of sugar
3 eggs
1/3 cup liquid honey
4 tbsp unsalted butter
5 to 6 cups unbleached flour
cornmeal for baking tray
1 egg white lightly beaten
sesame seeds or poppy seeds for decoration

Method

Sprinkle yeast on 1/2 cup of lukewarm water. Add sugar and stir to dissolve. Set aside until foamy. Beat together 3 whole eggs, honey, and butter. Add remaining 1 cup of lukewarm water. Blend in the yeast mixture and add 5 cups of flour. Beat for two minutes. Turn dough out and knead for five minutes. Add more flour as needed to make a smooth dough. Place in an oiled bowl to rise. Brush a little oil on the top of the dough and cover with a clean towel. Let rise in a warm place until doubled in size. Divide dough into 3 equal portions about 20 cm long. Pinch the three ropes together at one end then plait or braid together to form one loaf. Lightly oil a baking sheet and sprinkle with cornmeal. Place braided bread on this and cover with a towel. Let bread rise in a warm place until doubled in size. About 40 minutes. Heat oven to 160 degrees C. Brush the bread with egg white and poppy or sesame seeds. Bake until golden brown, 30 - 40 minutes. Cool on wire rack. Serve slices plain or with unsalted butter, fresh fruit jam or honey.

Use bread to make recipe for French toast in this book.

Health benefits of this recipe.

Honey's proven health benefits have been known for centuries for its natural healing and regenerative properties. (If you are allergic to honey, substitute maple syrup). Sesame seeds are high in iron and a good source of magnesium, potassium, folate and vitamin E and contain essential amino acids.

Jaq's Cracker Biscuits

Ingredients

1 1/2 cup buckwheat flour

1 tbsp poppy seeds

1/4 - 1/2 cup olive oil

cold water to mix

Method

Mix all ingredients together and add water to make a soft dough. Roll or pat onto a greased baking tray. Heat oven to 180 degrees C and bake crackers in one large piece until golden- about 20-30 minutes. Take care not to burn. Remove from the oven and cut into bars or squares. Store in airtight container. Serve with toppings as a snack or with soups as a bread replacement.

Variation

Vary the recipe by using different flours such as rye or whole-meal or corn, rice, oats. Experiment with half one flour and half another. Use other seeds like sesame, sunflower, and pumpkin. Add ground fresh nuts. Just be sure that all the ingredients are fresh. Store nuts and seeds in the freezer, to preserve freshness.

You can also add grated carrots and beetroot to this recipe and fresh herbs and make a denser, more cake like cracker.

Health benefits of this recipe.
Poppy seeds are high in potassium and zinc.

Applesauce Muffins

Ingredients

1 cup whole wheat flour

1 cup oats

1 tsp low-sodium baking powder

1/2 tsp baking soda

1 tsp cinnamon

1 cup unsweetened applesauce

1/2 cup low-fat milk

1/3 cup dark brown sugar

2 tbsp canola oil

1 large egg, lightly beaten

1/2 cup raisins

Method

Preheat oven to 200 degrees C. Lightly grease the bottom of a 12 cup muffin tin or use paper cases. Combine flour, oats, baking powder, baking soda and cinnamon together in a large bowl. In a small bowl mix applesauce, milk, sugar, oil and egg. Make a well in dry ingredients and add applesauce mixture. Stir until moist. Do not over mix. Add raisins. Fill muffin cups and bake for 20 minutes until cooked.

Blueberry and Orange Muffins

Ingredients

1 cup unbleached plain flour

1 cup whole wheat flour

1/2 cup raw sugar

1 tsp low-sodium baking powder

2 tbsp canola oil

1/4 cup orange juice

1 tsp vanilla extract

2 tbsp yogurt

1 egg

1 cup fresh blueberries or raspberries (or 1 cup frozen berries)

Method

Preheat oven to 200 degrees C. Mix flour, sugar, and baking powder together. In another bowl, mix oil, orange juice, vanilla, yogurt and egg together. Add this mixture to the flour mixture and stir gently just until moist. Do not over mix. Add raspberries or blueberries and fold in carefully. Do not beat. Fill a lightly greased 12-cup muffin tin. Bake 20 minutes or until cooked.

Blueberry Muffins

Ingredients

1 1/2 cup bran

1 cup non fat milk

1/2 cup unsweetened applesauce

1 egg

2/3 cup dark brown sugar

1 tsp pure vanilla extract

1/2 cup unbleached white flour

1/2 cup wholemeal flour

1/2 tsp baking soda

1 tsp low-sodium baking powder

1 cup blueberries, fresh or frozen

1 tsp cinnamon

Method

Preheat oven to 190 degrees C. Grease muffin tin. Mix together bran and milk. Leave to soak. In another bowl, mix applesauce, egg, sugar, and vanilla. Add bran mixture. Mix unbleached white flour, whole wheat flour, baking soda and baking powder together. Stir into bran mixture carefully. Gently fold in blueberries. Spoon into muffin cups. Bake 15 to 20 minutes until a skewer inserted in the middle comes out clean.

Poppy Seed Muffins

Ingredients

1 cup unbleached flour

1 cup whole-wheat flour

1/2 cup raw sugar

2 tbsp poppy seeds

1 1/2 tsp low-sodium baking powder

1/2 tsp baking soda

1 large egg

1 cup fat-free yogurt

1/4 cup canola oil

1/4 cup lime or lemon juice

1 tbsp lime or lemon zest

Method

Preheat oven to 200 degrees C. Mix dry ingredients together. Mix egg, yogurt, oil, lime or lemon zest, lime or lemon juice together. Make a well in the center of the dry ingredients and add the egg mixture. Do not over mix. Spoon into a lightly greased 12-cup muffin pan. Bake for 20 minutes.

Aromatic Essene Bread

Essene bread is a dense unbaked bread make of fresh sprouts. All the enzymes stay intact. An ancient recipe appears in the 1st century Aramaic manuscript when wafers were made from grain and water and cooked on sun heated stones. You can make and bake your own Essene bread and create a round flattened bread like a sweet moist dessert cake.

Method

Soak wheat berries (available from health food stores) and drain off the liquid. Sprout for two days in a dark place, rinse in cool water twice a day. Oil a meat grinder or nut mill/or food processor to stop the sprouts for sticking. Grind 2 cups of sprouts to make a sticky, juicy dough. Add nuts or dried fruits. Pre-soak fruit for 30 minutes in hot water and drain before adding to the dough 1/2 cup of chopped dates, or 1/2 cup dried apricots and/or 1/2 cup raisins. Add 1 tsp of cinnamon (optional). Wet your hands and shape the bread into a roll. Then shape it into a flat round loaf. Bake 1-2 hours at 120 degrees C. The outside of the bread should be firm but not hard. Cool on a cake rack. Can be frozen.

Cranberry Muffins

Ingredients

2 cups unbleached plain flour

1/2 cup raw sugar

1 tsp low-sodium baking powder

1 tsp ground cinnamon

1/2 tsp ground ginger

1/4 tsp ground nutmeg or mace

1 cup cooked pureed pumpkin

1 egg, beaten

1/4 cup canola oil

1 cup milk

1 cup fresh or frozen cranberries or dried cranberries roughly chopped

Method

Preheat oven to 180 degrees C. Mix flour, sugar, baking powder, spices. Combine pumpkin, egg, oil and milk in another bowl. Add pumpkin mixture to the flour mixture and stir until moist. Add cranberries. Fill muffin cups 2/3 full and bake for 20-30 minutes.

Pumpkin Muffins

Ingredients

1 1/2 cups unbleached plain flour

1 cup quick cooking oats

1/2 cup dark brown sugar

1/2 cup raisins

1 tsp low-sodium baking powder

1/2 tsp baking soda

1 tsp ground cinnamon

1/2 tsp ground nutmeg

1/2 tsp ground ginger

1/4 tsp ground allspice

1 cup cooked pumpkin

3/4 cup low fat milk

1/3 cup canola oil

1 egg lightly beaten

Method

Preheat oven to 190 degrees C. Line a 12-cup muffin tin with paper cases or grease the bottom of the tin lightly with oil. Combine dry ingredients. Combine pumpkin, milk, oil and egg. Beat well. Add the pumpkin mixture to the dry ingredients and stir until moist. Fill muffin tin 2/3 full and bake for 20-30 minutes until golden.

Banana Muffins

Ingredients

2 cups unbleached plain flour

1/2 cup raw sugar

2 tsp low-sodium baking powder

1/2 tsp baking soda

1 tsp ground cinnamon

1/4 tsp ground nutmeg or ground cardamom

1/4 cup canola oil

2/3 cup low fat milk

1 egg, lightly beaten

1 tsp vanilla

2 bananas, mashed

Method

Preheat oven to 180 degrees C. Lightly grease the bottoms of a 12-cup muffin pan. Mix flour, sugar, baking powder, baking soda, cinnamon and nutmeg together. Mix oil, milk, egg and vanilla together and add to the flour mixture. Stir until moist but do not over mix. Add mashed bananas and fold in gently. Fill muffins tins two-thirds full. Bake for 20 minutes.

Date Muffins

Ingredients

1 cup unbleached plain flour

1 cup whole wheat flour

1 tsp low-sodium baking powder

1/3 cup raw sugar

1 cup low fat milk

1/4 cup canola oil

1 tsp vanilla extract

2 eggs

1 apple, peeled, cored, finely chopped

1/2 cup finely chopped dates

Method

Preheat oven to 190 degrees C.
Lightly grease a 12-cup muffin pan with oil.
Mix flour, whole wheat flour, baking powder and
sugar together. Add milk, oil, vanilla, eggs and
stir. Do not over mix. Add apple and dates.
Fill muffin tins 2/3 full. Bake for 20 minutes.

Cherry muffins

Ingredients

1 cup unbleached plain flour

1 cup oats

1/2 cup raw sugar

2 tsp low-sodium baking powder

3/4 cup low fat milk

1 large egg, lightly beaten

1/4 cup canola oil

1 tsp almond extract

1 cup fresh or frozen cherries or 1/2 cup dried cherries, roughly chopped

Method

Preheat oven to 190 degrees C. Lightly grease a 12-cup muffin pan on the bottom, not the sides. Mix oats, flour, sugar, baking powder. Mix egg, milk, oil and almond extract in another bowl. Add this mixture into the flour mixture. Stir until moist. Fold in the cherries. Fill muffin cups 2/3 full. Bake 20 minutes.

Apricot muffins

Ingredients

1 1/2 cups unbleached plain flour

1/2 cup wheat germ

1/2 cup raw sugar

1 tsp low-sodium baking powder

1 tsp ground cardamom, ground aniseed or
ground ginger

1 cup low fat milk

2 tbsp canola oil

1 large egg

1/3 cup apricots or peaches, chopped (or use
dried apricots)

Method

Preheat oven to 190 degrees C.

Mix flour, sugar, baking powder and spice. Mix
milk, oil and egg.

Make a well in the middle of the flour mixture
and add egg mixture. Mix together but do not
over mix. Add apricots or peaches and fold in
carefully. Fill greased muffin cups 2/3 full. Bake
for 20 minutes.

Pineapple Muffins

Ingredients

1 1/2 cups of polenta (corn) flour

1 cup of plain flour

1 tsp low-sodium baking powder

1/4 cup sugar

1 cup unsweetened pineapple pieces

1 cup milk

2 eggs

2 tbsp unsalted butter, melted

2 tbsp honey or maple syrup

Method

Heat oven to 190 degrees C and grease muffin tins. Combine dry ingredients together. Combine eggs, milk, melted butter and golden syrup (or your choice of sweetener). Add to the dry ingredients. Add fruit. Stir just until combined. Do not over mix. Place in muffin tins and bake 15-20 minutes until cooked.

Oat Bran Muffins

Ingredients

1 cup unbleached plain flour

1 cup oat bran

1 tsp low-sodium baking powder

1 cup low fat milk

1/4 cup maple syrup

2 eggs

2 bananas, mashed

1 mango, chopped (or chopped apple)

Method

Preheat oven to 190 degrees C. Mix flour, oat bran and baking powder together. Place mashed banana, milk, maple syrup and eggs in a bowl and mix well. Add to the oat bran mixture and mix until just moist. Stir in apples and fill lightly greased muffin tins 2/3 full. Bake for 20-30 minutes until golden brown.

Wheat Germ Muffins

Ingredients

1 1/2 cups bran flakes

1/4 cup raw sugar

1 cup flour

1 tsp low-sodium baking powder

1 tbsp maple syrup or honey

1 cup milk

1 egg

1 cup fresh or frozen blueberries

Method

Heat oven to 190 degrees C and grease muffin tins. Combine dry ingredients together. Combine eggs and milk and melted butter and golden syrup. Add to the dry ingredients. Add blueberries. Stir just until combined. Do not over mix. Place in muffin tins and bake 15-20 minutes until cooked.

Carrot Muffins

Ingredients

2 cups whole meal flour

1 tsp low-sodium baking powder

1/4 cup wheat germ

1/4 cup unsweetened apple concentrate

3/4 cup unsweetened pineapple concentrate

2 egg whites

1 tsp vanilla essence

1/2 cup unsweetened crushed pineapple

1 cup finely grated raw carrot

Method

Heat oven to 190 degrees C and grease muffin tins. Combine flour, wheat germ together. Combine fruits and juices, egg whites, carrots and vanilla essence. Add to the dry ingredients. Stir just until combined. Do not over mix. Place in muffin tins and bake 15-20 minutes until cooked.

Pear Muffins

Ingredients

1 1/2 cups unbleached plain flour

1/2 cup whole wheat flour

1/4 - 1/2 cup raw sugar

1 tsp low-sodium baking powder

1 tsp cinnamon

1/2 tsp ginger

1/4 tsp nutmeg

3/4 cup low-fat milk

1 egg, beaten

2 tbsp canola oil

1 pear, peeled, cored and roughly chopped

Method

Preheat oven to 190 degrees C. Mix flour, sugar, baking powder and spices together. Mix milk, egg and oil together. Add milk mixture to flour mixture and stir until moist. Add chopped pear. Fill lightly greased muffin cups 2/3 full. Bake 20 minutes.

Berry Muffins

Ingredients

1 cup plain flour

1 1/2 cups wheat germ

1 tsp low-sodium baking powder

1/4 cup sugar

2 tbsp unsalted butter, melted

2 tbsp honey or maple syrup

1 cup milk

2 eggs

I cup raspberries or blueberries

Method

Heat oven to 190 degrees C and grease muffin tins. Combine dry ingredients together. Combine eggs and milk and melted butter and golden syrup (or your choice of sweetener). Add to the dry ingredients. Add fruit. Stir just until combined. Do not over mix. Place in muffin tins and bake 15-20 minutes until cooked.

Carrot Cake

Ingredients

1 1/2 cups unbleached plain flour

1/2 cup canola oil

1/2 cup dark brown sugar

1 cup chopped walnuts

1 cup grated carrots

1/2 low fat milk

3 eggs

1/2 tsp baking soda

1/2 teaspoon vanilla extract

1 1/2 tsp low-sodium baking powder

1/4 tsp ground cardamom

1 tsp ground cinnamon

1/4 tsp ground nutmeg

Method

Preheat oven to 175 degrees C. Grease and flour a 9 inch baking tin and line with baking paper. Sift the flour, baking soda, baking powder. Beat eggs with spices using a wire whisk. Stir in sugar and mix well. Beat in the oil and beat well. Add the flour mixture together with the milk to the egg mixture. Add carrots and walnuts. Pour into pan. Bake for 1 hour.

Spanish Orange and Almond Cake

Ingredients

4 large oranges

6 eggs

200g caster sugar

2 tablespoons lemon juice

1 teaspoon low-sodium baking powder

280g ground almonds

Method

Preheat oven to 180 degrees C. Cover oranges with cold water. Bring to the boil and simmer for 1 hour. Drain and leave until cold. Cut into quarters. Remove all seeds as they make the cake bitter. Process oranges to a pulp using a food processor. Add beaten eggs, sugar and lemon juice. Process for another minute. Add baking powder and ground almonds together. Mix again. Pour into a lightly greased 9 inch round cake tin. Bake 50 minutes until golden.

Walnut and Orange Cake

Ingredients

4 large eggs

2/3 cup raw sugar

1/2 cup canola oil

3/4 cup unbleached plain flour

3/4 cup semolina flour

1 1/2 tsp low-sodium baking powder

1 cup walnuts, finely chopped

1 tsp orange rind, finely grated

Ground cinnamon or cardamom

Coarsely chopped walnuts

Syrup

1/2 cup honey

1/2 cup water

1/2 tablespoon orange juice

1/2 tsp lemon juice

Method

First make the syrup: Stir honey, water, and lemon juice together and bring to a boil over high heat. Boil about 10 minutes until the syrup is reduced. Cool. Heat oven to 180 degrees C.

Lightly oil a 9 x 12 approx inch baking tin and dust with flour. Beat eggs and sugar until thick and pale. Slowly drizzle in oil and keep beating until blended. You can use a cake mixer on low speed for this. In another bowl mix flour, semolina, baking powder. Add this into the egg mixture and mix until combined. Stir in walnuts and lemon rind. Place in baking tin. Bake 30 or 35 minutes until golden. Using a toothpick make small holes in the cake when it comes out of the oven. Pour the syrup over the cake. Cool and remove from pan. Dust the top of the cake with cinnamon and sprinkle walnuts over.

Pilgrims Spoon Bread

Ingredients

3 cups milk

3/4 cup cornmeal

2 tbsp unsalted butter

2 eggs separated

1 tsp low-sodium baking powder

Method

Scald 2 cups of milk (almost to the boil). Add remaining milk and cornmeal. Cook 30 minutes. Stir often. Remove from heat. Add butter, egg yolks. Mix well. Add baking powder and mix. Fold in egg whites, stiffly beaten. Turn mixture into a well greased flat dish. Bake 30 minutes at 190 degrees C till golden brown.

Italian Cookies

Ingredients

1/2 cup whole raw hazelnuts

2 cups plain flour

1/2 cup granulated sugar

1 tsp low-sodium baking powder

1/2 cup raw almonds (whole)

3 tbsp unsalted butter

2 whole eggs

1 egg yolk

1 tsp vanilla extract

2 tsp freshly grated orange zest

Method

Preheat oven to 180 degrees C. Roast hazelnuts 15 minutes. Remove from oven. Cool remove skins. Place flour, baking powder, sugar in a bowl with nuts. Mix and add eggs, vanilla and orange zest. Mix ten minutes to make a soft dough. Divide dough into equal log shapes. Place logs on a greased baking paper and bake 10-15 minutes. When cool, slice thinly. Place the thin slices onto a baking tray lined with baking paper and bake again, just until light golden. Store in airtight jar or freezer.

Variation

Substitute pistachio nuts and add 1 tsp of ground anise instead of orange zest. Substitute orange zest for lime or lemon zest. Substitute pistachio nuts for hazelnuts.

Walnut Bars

Ingredients

3 eggs, well beaten

1/2 cup raw sugar

1 cup walnuts chopped

1 cup desiccated coconut

1 cup dates, chopped

3/4 cup wholemeal flour

1/4 cup wheat germ

Method

Heat oven to 180 degrees C. Combine all ingredients and mix well. Press down into a 9 inch square tin. Bake 20-30 minutes until golden and firm. Cut while warm into bars.

Apricot Squares

Ingredients

3 eggs, well beaten

1/2 cup raw sugar

1 cup shredded coconut

1 cup dried apricots or peaches, chopped

1/2 cup wholemeal flour

1/2 cup wheat germ

Method

Heat oven to 180 degrees C. Combine all ingredients and mix well. Press down into a 9 inch square tin. Bake 20-30 minutes until golden and firm. Cut while warm into squares.

Pecan Bars

Ingredients

3 eggs, well beaten

1/2 cup raw sugar

1 cup chopped pecan nuts

1 cup desiccated coconut

1 cup chopped dried cranberries

3/4 cup whole meal flour

1/4 cup wheat germ

Method

Heat oven to 180 degrees C. Combine all ingredients and press into a 9 inch tin. Bake for 20-30 minutes until golden. Cut while warm into bars.

Fig Bars

Ingredients

3 eggs, well beaten

1/2 cup raw sugar

1 cup chopped walnuts

1 cup desiccated coconut

3/4 cup chopped dried figs

1/4 cup chopped fresh pears

3/4 cup wholemeal flour

1/4 cup wheat germ

Method

Heat oven to 180 degrees C. Combine all ingredients and press into a 9 inch tin. Bake for 20-30 minutes until golden. Cut while warm.

Apple Bars

Ingredients

3 eggs, well beaten

1/2 cup raw sugar

1 cup chopped walnuts

1 cup desiccated coconut

3/4 cup raisins

1/4 cup chopped fresh apples

3/4 cup wholemeal flour

1/4 cup wheat germ

1 tsp cinnamon

Method

Heat oven to 180 degrees C. Combine all ingredients and press into a 9 inch tin. Bake for 20-30 minutes until golden. Cut while warm into bars.

Mr Chan's
Banana and Guava Bread

Ingredients

3 ripe bananas, mashed

1 tin of pink guavas, rinsed and drained, seeds removed, roughly chopped

1/2 cup brown sugar

2 eggs, lightly beaten

1 cup buttermilk

2 tbsp light vegetable oil or melted no-salt butter, cooled

2 cups organic unbleached self-raising flour

1/2 cup unbleached plain flour

1 tsp low-sodium baking powder

1/2 tsp cinnamon

Method

Heat oven to 170 degrees C. Mix bananas and guavas, sugar, egg, buttermilk and oil in a bowl. Sift flours, baking powder and cinnamon together. Add banana and guava mixture. Line a loaf pan 26 x 8 cm with baking paper and pour in mixture. Cook for 45-60 minutes until cooked. Test with a skewer. Makes a large moist loaf. Serve warm. Makes great toast.

ABOUT MENIERE MAN

This bestselling author is an Australian born writer and an award-winning Executive Creative Director, and partner in a successful advertising agency. At the height of his business career and aged just forty-six, he suddenly became acutely ill. He was diagnosed with Meniere's disease. He began to lose all hope that he would fully recover his health. However the full impact of having Meniere's disease was to come later. He lost not only his health, but his career and financial status as well.

It was his personal spirit and desire to get "back to normal" that turned his life around for the better. He decided that you can't put a limit on anything in life. Rather than letting Meniere's disease get in the way of life, he started to focus on what to do about getting over Meniere's disease.

With the advice on coping, healing, hope and recovery in his bestselling books, anyone reading the advice given, can make simple changes and find a way to get over Meniere's disease. As he went on to do.

These days life is different for the Author. He is a fit man who has no symptoms of Meniere's except for tinnitus and hearing loss in one ear. He does not take any medication. All the physical activities he enjoys these days require a high degree of balance: snowboarding, surfing, hiking, windsurfing, weightlifting, and riding a motorbike. All these things he started to do while suffering with Meniere's disease symptoms.

Meniere Man believes that if you want to experience

a marked improvement in health you can't wait until you feel well to start. You must begin to improve your health immediately, even though you may not feel like it.

With a smile and a sense of humor, the Author pens himself as Meniere Man, because Meniere's disease changed his life dramatically.

Today he is an author of twelve books including four Bestsellers and two #1 Bestsellers. He is a writer, painter, designer and exhibiting artist. He is married to a poet and essayist. They have two adult children. He spends his time writing and painting. He loves the sea, cooking, traveling, nature and the company of family, friends and his beloved dog.

ADDITIONAL INFORMATION

If you enjoyed this book and you think it could be helpful to others, please leave a review for the book.

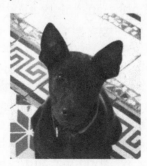

MENIERE MAN BOOKS

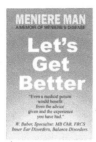

Let's Get Better
A Memoir of Meniere's Disease

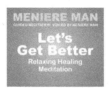

Let's Get Better CD
Relaxing & Healing Guided Meditation Voiced by
Meniere Man

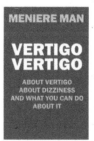

Vertigo Vertigo
About Vertigo About Dizziness and What You
Can Do About it

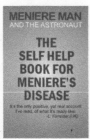

Meniere Man And The Astronaut
The Self Help Book for Meniere's Disease

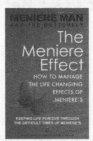

Meniere Man And The Butterfly
The Meniere Effect
How to Minimize the Effect of Meniere's on
Family, Money, Lifestyle, Dreams and You.

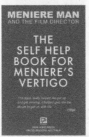

Meniere Man and the Film Director
The Self Help Book For Meniere's Vertigo

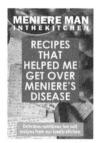

Meniere Man In The Kitchen.
Recipes That Helped Me Get Over Meniere's

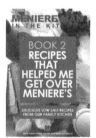

Meniere Man In The Kitchen.
Book 2

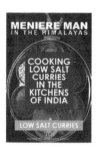

Meniere Man In The Himalayas.
Cooking Low Salt Curries In The Kitchens Of
India

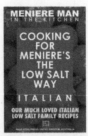

Meniere Man In The Kitchen. Cooking For Meniere's The Low Salt Way. ITALIAN

MENIERE SUPPORT NETWORKS

Meniere's Society (UNITED KINGDOM)
www. menieres.org.uk
Meniere's Society Australia (AUSTRALIA)
info@menieres.org.au
The Meniere's Resource & Information Centre (AUSTRALIA)
www.menieres.org.au
Healthy Hearing & Balance Care (AUSTRALIA)
www.healthyhearing.com.au
Vestibular Disorders association (AUSTRALIA
)www.vestibular .org
The Dizziness and Balance Disorders Centre (AUSTRALIA)
www.dizzinessbalancedisorders.com
Meniere's Research Fund Inc   (AUSTRALIA)
www.menieresresearch.org.au
Australian Psychological Society APS (AUSTRALIA)
www.psychology.org.au
Meniere's Disease Information Center (USA)
www.menieresinfo.com
Vestibular Disorders Association (USA)
www.vestibular.org
BC Balance and Dizziness Disorders Society (CANADA)
www.balanceand dizziness.org
Hearwell (NEW ZEALAND)
www.hearwell.co.nz
WebMD.
www.webmd.com
National Institute for Health
www.medlineplus.gov
Mindful Living Program
www.mindfullivingprograms.com
Center for Mindfulness
www. umassmed.edu.com

Shopping Essentials

Kelp - Flakes, granules, dried, Powder
Arrowroot -
Raw sugar
Wholemeal Flour
wheatgerm
Cranberries

Printed in March 2024
by Rotomail Italia S.p.A., Vignate (MI) - Italy